Practicing Tai Chi

Ways to Enrich Learning for Beginning and Intermediate Practitioners

By Paul Tim Richard

Published by Paul T. Richard Writings
ISBN-13: 978-0692132104 (Custom Universal)
ISBN-10: 0692132104
BISAC: Health & Fitness / Exercise

Paultrichard.wordpress.com

Cover photo by Paul T. Richard

CONTENTS

"That martial arts are a system of self-defense is self-evident, and the medical benefits of martial exercise [are] not a great leap. However, Chinese culture has taken the martial arts several steps further, merging them with meditation and inner alchemy, and finally presenting them as a path of ultimate self-realization through the Tao."

(Wile, Douglas, Lost T'ai-Chi Classics from the Late Ch'ing Dynasty, 1996.)

Acknowledgements

I am grateful to all with whom and from whom I've learned. Master Susan A. Matthews, MS, ND, ushered me into the taijiquan world and introduced me to Master George Xu (Xu Guo Ming) of Shanghai, China and San Francisco, California. Both have placed me into a position of learning I found challenging and daunting in a slow, often painful, path of change.

Their efforts helped me to overcome my self-inflicted resistance to learning. Even though I accepted the challenge in my own way, I cannot say I did my best, or even do my best now. I dare to say, however, that I strove and still strive to be better than yesterday.

I thank my fellow learners over the years in various workshops, seminars and annual camps—too many to name. I am grateful particularly for my students who have accepted the challenge themselves and with whom I travel the path of learning, with whom I've spent hours discussing and practicing tai chi's subtler energies. I learn from them as much as I hope they learn from me.

I thank those first practitioners of Old China for their discoveries, diligence and wherewithal to pass their knowledge on to subsequent generations who carried it onward. Now, practitioners across the world are discovering the gift. Although we retain only a fraction (I'm told) of what once was known, it is a powerful remnant for us to take forward on a journey of rediscovery.

What This Book Is About

Practicing Tai Chi represents experience gathered across two decades of learning and doing tai chi and qigong. Much of it is drawn from my course: "The Fundamentals of Tai Chi." It is also drawn from topics I blog about, such as what tai chi is, why do it, how to do it and, importantly, how to think about integrating it into daily life.

It's about living tai chi and about just being in the moment, in the flow. It's about being aware, being observant, being still in motion, yet active in stillness. It's about being open to discovery, about recognizing accomplishment, about sharing with others, about being of pure heart, open mind, strong body, and free spirit.

What you'll read in this text falls somewhere between practicalities and theory. It is personal in tone, yet universal in nature. Practical refers to basic tai chi movements. You develop a routine of moving in specific ways. Practice helps to enhance awareness as we train our powers of observation to become sharper, quicker and accurate.

Much that you'll read is about change in that you have to change something about the way you move. That means to actually change your position, to shift your weight, to feel the difference in the position of a muscle or tendon, perhaps a bone or joint, compared to another. You'll find techniques for practice along these lines.

Tai chi theory is more involved if you're unfamiliar with the basics. The theory comes in after enough training has been achieved. In *Practicing Tai Chi*, I offer a number of concepts and ideas for understanding tai chi in a broader theoretical context to apply in practice.

I'm also interested in how an individual experiences tai chi. The interface of where the individual meets a practice is where discovery and accomplishment take place. This is where the known meets the unknown, the yet-to-be discovered—where all the action and adventure takes place. Tai chi is a personal experience that can be shared and that's what I do in *Practicing Tai Chi*.

Who This Book Is For

With so many people seeking alternatives for healthy living, demand is increasing for information about tai chi as a complementary activity for cultivating health and well-being. In *Practicing Tai Chi*, you can find tips for getting the best out of tai chi. Perspectives on how to think about a tai chi practice are offered to help develop a home practice and stimulate new avenues of learning.

Learners who have already begun tai chi and have some knowledge of its basics will probably learn a lot from this book. Whether you've practiced for some time or very little, if you feel ready to move into a higher level of understanding about tai chi, then I believe you will find useful insights.

I wrote *Practicing Tai Chi* for learners in my classes and to share with others. Many learners who begin learning with me are absolute beginners who have had little idea of what tai chi is. So I think of this book as a reference guide for concepts and activities to help build a strong and knowledgeable practice.

Much of what I discuss is not commonly known by the average tai chi practitioner. If you have studied the tai chi classics and history, or studied in-depth with acknowledged masters of Chinese Internal Martial Arts, then some of it will sound familiar, albeit with a personal slant based on my own particular experience and studies.

I believe that we all need a self-discovery. Every day that you practice what you learned in tai chi class is a new exploration, blazing trail in new landscapes. The landscape in this case is the self. If you're into self-discovery, then I hope my book will work for you.

Who Should Do Tai Chi?

As an exercise, the health benefits of doing tai chi are strong reasons for anyone to choose to learn it. You don't need to be an expert to feel the effects of doing tai chi. Knowing even a little can help to improve other kinds of activities that involve movement: walk, run, swim, dance, lift, ride a horse, ride a bicycle, sit, climb, stand. If you engage in any of these, I encourage exploring the transferability of tai chi skills.

Tai chi may not be for everyone because you may not be ready for it. It takes focus, concentration and some effort. Even though the master says tai chi should be effortless ("minimum effort, maximum result"), real tai chi takes concentration. The good thing is it gets easier, more familiar, more comfortable with practice.

What kind of person wants to learn tai chi? A person who:

- needs/wants more physical activity
- needs/wants more mental focus
- is healing from injury
- wants to do more than an occasional fitness class
- enjoys interacting with others in an educational setting
- wants to delve deeper in the study of the subject
- is looking for a practice that complements other activities
- is having health issues, such as autoimmune disease.
- is having balance issues.
- is interested in martial arts
- wants to delve deeper into self-awareness
- wants a moving meditation, as opposed to sitting meditation
- is feeling stressed and wanting a relaxation practice
- is interested in making new friends

CHAPTER ONE

A (personal) philosophy of learning

"...Although the Dao or the Way has always existed in eternity and rigorously conforms to precise laws, it must always be discovered for oneself. It is always new. One must always struggle to free oneself from the spell of thoughts and images that at best reflect only what has been experienced in the past."
(Gia-Fu Feng and Jane English, translators.
Tao Te Ching, 1972, p85.)

Let's start at "a" beginning, rather than at "the" beginning. With a subject as amorphous and historically lengthy as taijiquan you can start anywhere and still find yourself only at *a* beginning.

Taijiquan has been described as having developed in three areas of study and practice:

- form practice;
- technique and fighting applications, often in two-person push hands practice; and,
- theory and philosophy.

I pay a lot of attention to philosophy based on personal perspectives that arise from my practice. Without practice, however, you wouldn't be doing tai chi. You have to do it to know it.

Most beginners learn tai chi by memorizing moves and sequences of moves (forms) which, for many, takes considerable effort at first. It's achievable, though.

For me, the question of how to learn tai chi often supersedes the question of how to do it — "learning how to learn," in other words. A look into the learning process, or the experience of learning, itself may offer a deeper insight into why we do tai chi; definitely into *how* we do tai chi.

Learning tai chi is a process of continual growth in skill and knowledge.

Each practitioner is always engaging in the activity of learning itself. Not from the perspective in which the student needs the teacher's help, which is "handed down to him" (Zull, 2002, p. xiii). Actual learning takes place in the brain and in the body, not in the relationship between teacher and student. So the question of how to learn tai chi, asked by the learner, stimulates a new dynamic. Tai chi is the teacher.

Learning tai chi is a process of continual growth in skill and knowledge. It is a matter of sharpening our powers of observation and cultivating greater awareness of the manner in which we move. It also creates opportunities to cultivate insight into one's self. I've learned that we are not the same learners as when we begin, and we will not remain the same as long as we continue practice.

Tai chi practice allows practitioners to tap into a creative side in ways that, often enough, are lost to a vast swath of humanity. We're all naturally creative, but we're inhibited by forces in our lives, often external, but often enough from within as we inhibit ourselves.

We're advised to live in the present moment, but how do you experience a moment more fully—or at least to any degree beyond what we are normally cognizant of feeling? For most, that's a fraction of our inherent capability. Whether or not you're clear of your what, how, and why of tai chi, it matters that you try, if only to cultivate a clearer sense of being in the present moment.

So often, once we have been on a path of learning something unfamiliar, such as tai chi and qigong, we encounter resistance. The practical part of tai chi is key to meeting that resistance within ourselves with equanimity and wisdom.

One must have a reason to do tai chi, not just that you have to do it, or that someone holds your feet to the fire to make sure you do what you're told. You want to freely choose to practice and feel satisfied that you have.

Still, we often force ourselves if no one else does, and call it discipline. For me there are two kinds of discipline. One, is doing what we know is good for us and what we have committed to do despite not feeling like it. Discipline is also when you meet adversity (when things don't go as expected) with serenity. Tai chi helps you cultivate such serenity. Regardless of your definition of discipline, after making effort, we are eventually happy we did.

Tai chi is not about making it happen,
but letting it happen.

The Four Gifts: Life, Breath, Awareness, and Mobility

Humans receive four gifts at birth (at least) without which we cannot live. Too many of us lose a great opportunity by not examining these mysteries in some organized manner, consciously and deliberately. Tai chi can help open our awareness to these gifts that make up our whole being. For me, a tai chi practice offers a chance to tap back into them and renew our connection with them.

Life

The first is life. Nobody knows why the heart beats. Why wonder about things we don't understand? We go through life immersed in all sorts of goings on without pondering why the heart beats and keeps on beating and beating while we do what we do with little to no regard for it. Through tai chi and qigong, we turn our attention towards our life force, or our *Qi (Chi)*, with the intention of enhancing it and becoming more conscious and familiar with it.

Breath

Breath underlies every movement we make. To move from here to there, a tai chi practitioner uses awareness of breath, body position and intention to travel from here to there, from this step to that, from this position to that position. Breath is a vehicle by which we live. Applying breath and movement in tai chi practice is a foundational activity that you (have to) do before everything else.

Awareness

Our senses demonstrate awareness. We see, hear, feel, smell, taste. I always think I'm missing one. I'm sure there are more we are not aware of. Deep within, from a silent part of us, we are aware of everything. It is ancient, timeless and vast, beyond day and night, light and dark. It seems to sleep while we move through life, going places, doing things, saying things, thinking things, being things. But we've just forgotten it's there. Taiji is a means of acknowledging it, listening to it, reconnecting with it, moving it and moving with it.

Mobility

We have been given the gift of mobility. Mobility distinguishes us from many other beings on Earth. The quality of our movement distinguishes us even further. Mobility has been a real instrument in human survival. Tai chi practice takes this ability to conscious levels.

These four gifts make up the foundation of our lives. Taking them into account as a foundational part of tai chi will enhance your practice. Internal martial arts practice is a way to treat them with reverence. With awareness of them we can learn to preserve our beings and maintain optimum functionality in our mind, body and spirit through conscious, deliberate movement—better mobility, heart function, circulation, digestion, metabolism, and so on.

CHAPTER TWO

What, Why, and How of Tai Chi

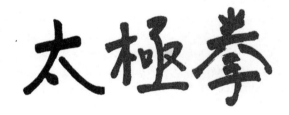

What is Tai Chi?

Tai chi can be any number of things for any number of people. This is one reason why it has so much appeal to diverse communities of interest. Tai chi is a true gift to the human race, a great discovery.

For me, tai chi is first and foremost a movement practice in its simplest form. I call it *art of internal movement*. I discuss this throughout the book.

In some aspects, tai chi is a mood that you experience, then cultivate and mature over time. You "internalize" the mood of tai chi more and more as you practice it. For example, a sense of both stillness and movement becomes more present when you're not actually in a practice session.

In more-mature stages of learning, tai chi is a precise art. You probably won't be that precise when you're still new to it and learning to adapt your body and mind to practice. But as you gain insights into the quality of your movement and in the nature of movement in general, the mental processes of observation and awareness building mature. Through practice you see your movements in new ways.

The point at which learning occurs is when new things are encountered and recognized, and where known things are grasped in new ways.

Tai chi is an art of change, or of adaptability. Change can be like the shifting of a scale as it balances itself. Weight placed on one side of the scale produces an equal and opposite reaction on the other side. The human body, from a tai chi perspective, is continuously attempting to balance itself, seeking equilibrium on many levels in response to forces exerted upon it. This takes place whether we are conscious of it or not, from the external to the internal, the superficial to the profound, from the surface to the depths, from the grand to the minuscule, the outer to the inner.

I could continue on ridiculously, but conscious tai chi practice is this kind of journey—from the outer realms of your body to the inner, from the broader states of awareness to deeper states of cognition. You are the artist engaged in the art of adapting and changing to shifts of the scale.

Tai chi can become a "way of life." Its defining principle is always active whether in practice or in daily living. Your perspective shifts as new information is presented and you adapt and become more skilled at tai chi *and* life.

You also see older information in fresh ways. This could be in the form of difficulties, sudden events, news, whether good or bad, things you see happen to others, and myriad possibilities that life reveals. This is part of the learning process and the process of living.

Tai chi is listening to your body and doing what it tells you. Listening and following through. Listening possesses a quality of not listening, letting something happen of its own accord and not working hard at it, or disrupting its process of unfolding.

This sort of meditation is one of focusing attention on a locus in the body and a specialized movement, or pattern of moves, and sustain that focus for an extended period of time.

Tai chi is often referred to as a "moving meditation," but, for me, it's also a path to a meditative state. It's a meditation on movement while in the act of moving. This sort of meditation is one of focusing attention on a locus in the body and a specialized movement, or pattern of moves, and sustain that focus for an extended period of time.

The manner and depth in which you concentrate informs how you move, which in turn provides insights into a variety of things, such as your posture and balance, where you have unnecessary tension, how and where you carry stress, what your habits of movement are and whether they are beneficial, or whether they need to be replaced by new modes of motion.

Tai chi and qigong are therapeutic practices. They are forms of self-therapy, or even self-hypnosis in which you can enter a kind of trance. However, the process of focusing attention on specific tasks and maintaining concentration on them goes beyond a trance-like state of being, by placing the activity itself at the forefront of our attention. You have to stay conscious to do that.

Tai chi is a great way to orient yourself within your environs. I practice in nature regularly, along lakes and streams, on mountain tops, valleys, even roadsides, cities, …wherever I am, actually. It engages the senses in being present in the moment. It helps me get a feel for a place, and situates me within it, giving me a more tangible sense of life and existence. I feel more alive.

Tai chi is something you do yourself for yourself. It is not a pill you take then sit back and let it do its thing. You have to be engaged. Memory, repetition, study … go into it. Tai chi works best when you immerse into it.

What you give attention to is key. What you focus on is what you are working on. Everything else is taken care of automatically.

In beginning tai chi, you're teaching your body to do things that it doesn't normally do. As a child you moved naturally; your body was new and unimpeded. But with aging we learn to move incorrectly. This is especially brought on by neglect to the inner workings of our bodies. More-efficient, natural, movement is called for.

Tai chi produces more-natural movements, as opposed to what has become habitual movement. When you're doing tai chi movement, you're realigning and rebalancing bones, joints, ligaments, and tendons. You're essentially massaging organs, too. You're also moving the lymphatic system, a process which transports toxins out of the body. You're pumping freshly oxygenated blood to the cells. I could go on, but this gives a picture. Tai chi movement does all kinds of good stuff for you.

Similarly, your mental processes get a workout. You're stretching your mind beyond its usual limits. We all know how to do this. We just need to be exposed to it again.

What is "Internal"?

As I mention earlier, three categories for exploration in taijiquan are: form practice; technique and fighting, and; theory and philosophy. Many practitioners, if not most, incorporate all three, but also focus on a thread that runs through them all: the internal.

Taijiquan is usually referred to as an "internal" martial art. Internal is a major focus in my *Fundamentals* course, as well as this book. It's a

broad term that covers a number of practices and principles for applying in movement. You can journey deeply into the question of
what internal is and how you can access it in practice.

The topic of internal as it was introduced to me by my teachers was,
at first, just words to me—two dimensional references to a phenome-
non of which I had had no experience. Internal? _Qi?_ Life force? Spiral energy? Terminology piled up around me as I worked on understanding.

At first, my grasp lacked depth, experience and awareness. But as I
amassed skill and experience, I came to describe internal for myself as
the more intricate, deeper levels of movement that you train to narrow your focus down to. It's not a single thing, but a combination of
principles and practices that you can learn and internalize. It goes
from the practical and corporeal to the more abstract and esoteric.

This practice always leads the attention to the most minute motion
deep in your being, not just your physical body, which is usually the
focus in the beginning of practice. But you also have your mind, your
_Yi_ (意), your spirit (S_hen_—神) , and your _Qi_ (气), or life force energy,
upon which you can train your attention.

At some point, regularly and sincerely focusing attention on deeper
levels triggers changes in the quality of your movements. Your move
may become bigger or smaller, or more power may come with it. It's
exponential, as in what I've heard my teacher, George Xu, say often:
"minimum effort, maximum result."

Immerse more fully by enhancing your powers of observation. Perception and cognition can lead to meaning and understanding.
Sooner or later, with enough practice, you can arrive at a point of
asking how you may go deeper into the question of what internal is
and how you can access it in practice.

This idea defies what average people usually think. If your long-held
thinking has grown static, shallow, and relies on unexamined assumptions you'll have difficulty picking up on the more intrinsic details of

taijiquan. Understanding this boils down to being free in your movement so that you will adjust to the constant flux of the energy of being alive.

You'll read this a few times in this book: Let the mind picture the move before you move at all, then let the vital energy move your body. I'm simply referring to the "life force" that practitioners try to connect with. You're not just learning moves and sets of moves. You're learning how to be alive in the present moment. You're learning how to feel the energy in any given moment.

Sometime ago, Master George Xu opened up a small door in my imagination when he described an aspect of the Taiji Tu—the *Yin-Yang* symbol—which depicts *Yin* is in *Yang* and *Yang* is in *Yin*. One is embedded in the other, symbolizing depth. Plus, it's three-dimensional. *Yin-Yang* motion can go deeper inside of you, not just happen on the surface.

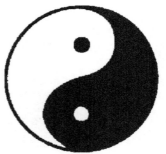

In another dynamic, when *Yang* reaches its ultimate expression it transforms into *Yin*, and when *Yin* achieves its ultimate expression, it becomes *Yang*. And so it goes perpetually. We actually replicate this dynamic in motion.

To take the analogy even further: In one dimension, one's focus deepens and narrows. Extraneous details are shed. The distracting concerns of daily life are shunted to a place of less significance. Stress levels that generate physical and emotional tension, which can lead to illness and, often enough, psychological disorders, are eventually lessened with practice.

In another dimension, the attention widens and expands. Your mind is open, expansive. Your body feels a sensation of being a wide-mouthed receptacle of insight and energy well beyond the defined edges of your physicality.

You can perceive both of these dimensions of awareness separately or simultaneously. You can practice one at a time in the early stages of your training. With experience you will be practicing multiple dimensions at the same time: remembering steps in the form sequence, visualizing moving using mind intent and feeling, or sensing the flow of energy and directing it.

Keep these things in mind as you read this book and as you practice. The question of what tai chi is never ends because it is alive, responsive and vibrant. Every time you practice, you redefine it for yourself into a clearer view. You never arrive at all-knowing. Change lies at the heart of practice. Even if you knew exactly what moving meditation means, it doesn't encompass the full scope of discoveries that the practice of tai chi can have for the individual practitioner.

The what of tai chi can be described in many more ways than these I list here. Each practitioner can share views unique to their own experience. These that I share represent a few of my own that I hope draw a picture of what tai chi can be for you.

An Analogy for "Internal"

The body is a vessel that contains 70% water, blood, lymph. I like the word vessel. It suggests a container that holds something, but also one that travels through space, carrying its contents along. The human body is such a vessel. One way to perceive motion when doing tai chi is to intend moving the contents, not the hard-edged structure that holds the contents. Move the liquid, not the container. This softens the edge and you can sense going outside of yourself.

Why Do Tai Chi?

There are as many reasons to do tai chi as there are people practicing. I list reasons that go beyond the conventionalized reasons, such as balance, circulation, relaxation, and disease management.

The points I make here are really my own, but I think they offer insights into why someone else may want to do tai chi that are more personal in nature compared to the usual reasons that you read about.

I believe that people turn to tai chi because they intuit a missing link in themselves and they want to get it back. They want to reconnect with their natural selves.

Normally, we develop only as far as necessary to function within our milieu to meet the demands of everyday living. As we age, some of us realize that this approach has squelched inherent parts of us and our natural abilities. This shows in the reduced range of motion that we see in older age. Recognizing the discrepancy, we want to correct it; so we begin looking for ways to do that. Some of us discover tai chi and qigong.

So when someone asks why do tai chi, my answer often is that we're trying to return to our natural selves. We're trying to return to our natural abilities that we had when we were younger. What are those natural abilities? They are our natural ability to learn using cognition and the senses, and to build upon what is learned.

With tai chi, we can enhance our senses through conscious, deliberate use. It's a form of self-improvement that rewards the effort to learn in a multitude of ways that lead to an overall sense of well-being and more energy, self-assuredness and even confidence.

Doing tai chi and qigong helps to relieve some symptoms of serious ailments, such as autoimmune illnesses like Parkinson's Disease, fibromyalgia, arthritis of all kinds, muscular sclerosis, scoliosis. Indeed, researchers in various science fields are only recently turning more rigorous attention to the subject with surprising findings.

Increasingly, published reports confirm and affirm the efficacy of tai chi and qigong at helping to reduce symptoms of many common ailments, even possibly addressing their causes. Anxiety, chronic pain, including back pain, depression, acute-injury healing, even obesity, are all part of the long and seemingly growing list of ailments that tai chi and qigong, to some degree, seem to affect positively.

In one National Institutes of Health-funded report (http://www.arthritis.org/about-arthritis/types/back-pain/articles/tai-chi-low-back-pain.php), researchers found that more patients spent money on treating lower back pain than some 14 other conditions examined in the study.

Another study (http://www.spine-health.com/wellness/yoga-pilates-tai-chi/tai-chi-posture-and-back-pain) in Australia reports that tai chi is good for improving posture and alignment. It states that, "Practicing Tai Chi may therefore reduce the practitioner's back pain through application." This speaks to the concept of *zhong ding* in tai chi practice, which I discuss further on.

These are just examples of what's out there to read and learn from. The National Institutes of Health and the Center for Complementary and Integrative Health are prime sources for dozens of reports.

Reported health results are motivation enough to learn tai chi. But actual practitioners know that we feel differently after practice. We know that results accumulate over time into a repertory of greater skill and potential.

At least some of tai chi's efficacy comes from its meditative qualities. Slowing your mind and body down, moving attentively and breathing fully, you become more sensitive and aware of changes within you and around you. Tai chi practice helps to cultivate sensitivity to subtle changes in the body and beyond.

If you're interested in this ability, then you should practice tai chi. It has implications for overall health and well-being, because you should be more able to detect shifts in your physical conditions early and possibly avoid some illnesses.

For example, you could feel the first signs of a cold early on, and slow or even stop its development. This sounds like a big claim, but more evidence is being published about the preventative nature of tai chi, particularly when it comes to chronic issues that arise with aging and injury.

Years ago, in my early fifties I got shingles, which can be painful and, for some, last a long time. For me, it lasted about two weeks and was relatively mild. I attribute that to recognizing it and seeing a doctor and getting medication practically the first day I detected something odd. I attribute that decision, as well as my quick recovery, to my tai chi practice. These are only some reasons to look into tai chi as a health maintenance and preventative practice.

Ways to Think About Tai Chi Practice

In class, I talk about "places" to get to in tai chi practice—milestones in developing skill, such as *see-feel-do*, whole body moves as a single unit, being "connected," being "weighted in gravity," feeling the *qi* go through, freeing the muscle.

You might think, "Wow, these things sound cool, but how am I going to get there?" I describe these milestones so you'll know what you're working towards, but also be more likely to recognize them when you come across them for the first time in your practice.

Change

What is tai chi good for? For one thing, as a method for making change happen, such as breaking "bad" habits we don't want anymore. For most of us, changing a habit is not as easy as just saying you will.

Actually, from a tai chi perspective, we don't break a habit as much as redirect our attention to learning a practice that makes doing the old, undesirable habit pointless and useless. We don't break a habit; we choose to do something else. That's where tai chi comes in. In tai chi and qigong, you learn a skill that makes you feel better; thus the habit that you wish to lose, loses its importance and fades away.

Keep in mind that it takes effort on your part and learning how to recognize change. It could be that you realize your alignment is out of balance and you find that you can shift your posture a little one way or another, and you feel a little relief from that ache in your lower back. Or maybe your sinuses will clear up and you will have fewer allergy episodes.

Change takes place in an energetic sense. Tai chi makes energy available to us once again by redirecting the energy spent on unwanted practices towards doing what helps us to feel better, more contented, more alive. Through tai chi practice, we actually build a memory of feeling better. When bad things happen we are more capable of recalling that feeling, which strengthens our resolve.

Here are some synonyms for change that have practical applications in a tai chi practice. For example, alter or alternate moves. Shift weight. Modify a pattern. Do a move differently somehow. Adjust your force. And so on.

Alter	Vary
Shift	Modify
Redefine	Transform
Differ	Fluctuate
Adjust	

In a broader perspective, tai chi practice can lead to changes in the perception of one's self. The personal experience of taijiquan is where the greatest chance for growth within larger contexts of life exists. When each person grows, we all do. As my teacher once said, "You want to change the world? Change yourself." Similarly, "all change is self-change." I fancy that change means to adapt in order to become more aware of an infinitely more encompassing power than the individual self.

Experience Tai Chi

Many people don't actually know what real tai chi is. In order to, you have to "experience" it for yourself. Looking at tai chi as an experience helps it look less like work, or like the proverbial bad-tasting medicine the doctor orders you to take. You know it's supposed to be good for you, but you don't do it anyway.

Experiencing tai chi takes time—of which most of us seem to have little. What do you do about that? It's simple…make time. Every time I practice, I discovery new things about my body, how I move and don't move, and about my mind and my life force.

You have to do it to get a clear understanding. Not only that; most everyone will agree that if you do tai chi, you *will* feel different even the first time you take a class. In fact, the whole measure of tai chi is whether you feel the difference after an hour or two of practice. Bottom line: you should. Even a minute or two of deep, authentic effort will produce a feeling of well-being and health.

Integrating Tai Chi in a Busy Life in a Busy World

For many practitioners, or would-be learners, learning tai chi takes time out of your busy day. You have to go to a class, learn moves, remember them, then practice them to internalize them.

Doing that as part of a daily routine becomes less time sensitive once you know what to practice on your own. I see the issue as a "timing" thing. If we time it right, we can do tai chi anytime we wish by simply recognizing that we have a minute or two to do something—however little it is (see "timing" later on).

It's also a question of what kinds of movement can fall under the category of "tai chi." It's easy to know what that is. I give learners several things they can do and they can be practicing intricate subtle principles of tai chi anytime they think of it.

The challenge is to shift the mind from the demands of work to tai chi even for just a minute or two. That's the issue, not whether we have time or not. There always is time.

Whether it's having time, not having time, or simply, timing, doing tai chi is one challenge. Having energy is perhaps a greater, deeper challenge. Yet, ironically, having practiced enough tai chi generates energy. Rather, it releases stuck *qi* that movement makes available to you. This is energy that you were born with and returns to you once freed up—like a homing pigeon returns to the roost. Recall the energy you had when you were a child. Do you think you could ever get it back? Maybe, maybe not, but you can begin now and I believe you'll get some of it back.

I see the issue as a "timing" thing. If we time it right, we can do tai chi anytime.

Get Familiar, Get Comfortable, Refine

Learning the simplest things in tai chi can be a challenge at first; not because they're difficult, but because we're unfamiliar with them. For example, sometimes new learners grasp the details of simple cloud hands only with significant effort. Or we have to remind ourselves over and over to remember to maintain a proper stance while moving the upper body.

With practice though, we gradually build familiarity with the moves, then we become more comfortable, then we can refine what we've learned. Every successive move is a refinement of the previous one. Over time, with continued focus, we improve at the process of learning itself. We are able to sustain concentration longer and with more depth.

Minimum Effort

I know I say that tai chi takes time to learn, but that's not quite accurate. It takes "effort" and, over time, you gain a greater depth of understanding, knowledge and skill; all of which in turn produce greater benefits beyond what a beginner might experience. Effort, in this case, doesn't mean hard work or strenuous activity. It means doing easy moves easily, so to speak. Being relaxed but active, calm, alive.

Minimum effort means that each movement is performed with as little force as possible. Force refers to physical effort, usually more than is needed to accomplish a task. Minimum effort allows us to shift our unexamined habit away from the physical and to help quieten the body so we can feel and listen to our life force. This is what tai chi and qigong are really about. Listening to *qi* and the subtle energies that we are capable of tapping into, and that produce some powerful results with minimum effort once we know what we're looking for.

Know your limits, learn what they are, then go beyond them.
It could be physical, mental, emotional.
You are more resilient than you think.

Feeling Overwhelmed

Beginners sometimes feel overwhelmed by the amount of information they're suddenly exposed to, at least the way I teach it. Sometimes, a person will think he has to get it all at once, which often feels like much too big of a challenge, so he doesn't practice. I tell them don't expect yourself to know it all at once.

No one starts out knowing all there is to know. No one is perfect from the beginning, at least in the perfect execution of the moves and postures. The allure of tai chi is to refine and perfect. To practice. If you can't do a move, don't let it be an excuse not to try anyway, anywhere, anytime. Get familiar with them, get comfortable with them, then refine them each time you begin another session.

In other words, just keep doing the moves. Work on exercises learned in class, such as single-basic moves and qigong, visualizations and form. Try to remember something. Even if you work on only one thing, work on it. This is key to getting going. Set up a time and place to practice, even if it's for five minutes.

You probably have heard coaches in the past say you have to be motivated and committed in order to be successful. You need discipline. I'm not so sure that applies exactly the same way in tai chi practice, although it might sound applicable to some degree. Discipline means to do something even when we don't feel like it. I would say that if you are experiencing resistance, then do a little bit, not a lot, to prove to yourself that you can overcome inertia or laziness or procrastination.

Commitment seems to require a more-developed mindset than motivation. Commitment is probably not the most accurate word for the image I have, which is one more like feeling a need for nourishment—to nourish one's self through practice and study. To meditate or contemplate or ponder how to satiate and sustain a state of being, or a mood, that one may carry, or be carried by.

This relates to enhancing awareness and perspective. Shedding preconceived notions of what a practice is or should be is one of the fields of discovery for the seeker of nourishment.

Limitations and Self-Imposed Limitations

I describe two concepts encountered in tai chi practice by beginners and intermediates: limitations and self-imposed limitations. Limitations are conditions that stunt the ability to do tai chi. For example, we might have an injury that limits the range of motion of the knee. Knee replacements seem to have a limited ranged of mobility.

In contrast, "self-imposed limitations" are boundaries we place on ourselves. We don't want to stretch the hamstring muscles because it's uncomfortable, or maybe we're afraid we'll hurt ourselves. That could be a legitimate assessment and, ultimately, only you can decide if it's accurate and fair. But be aware that we limit ourselves by telling ourselves we can't do something. In fact, we actually could despite what we tell ourselves.

We may not be able to do much about limitations and we may be able to do more with self-imposed limitations, but both are merely boundaries that can be expanded, or even dissolved, with practice. Finding the balance between the two extremes is key to progress.

CHAPTER THREE

Developing Your Practice

"Change your mind to change your body. Practice Gongfu to understand your body and your life."

Practice at home as soon as you begin learning tai chi. Solo practice is essential to the overall practice of tai chi, along with group practice and private lessons with a master practitioner. Developing a solo practice is really a matter of getting information and utilizing it to help shift routines. Tai chi itself provides that information and nurtures positive change.

Even though promoters, myself included, often say tai chi is simple and easy, beginners often don't practice between classes. Tai chi can be challenging, as well as easy. There are a number of reasons for not practicing. One is that a novice doesn't really have a lot of information and knowledge upon which to build a practice. More accurately, I find that beginners don't see the value and applicability of the information they are getting from group class and the teacher. Another reason is that most people have a daily routine that tai chi has yet to find a place in. Finding space for it takes some effort for the beginner.

All excuses aside—too busy, lazy, no time, hard to break old habits, lack of confidence, or some other form of resistance—one reason lies deeper below the surface of the usual excuses.

We are challenged at some level of awareness. If we can accept that this happens and become familiar with how it plays out in our daily routines, then we might be better able to overcome this common obstacle ... this opponent. Your own resistance is an opponent, faking you, coming after you, throwing you off balance.

"You don't have to be the best,
just be better than yesterday."

What is a "Practice"?

It can be simpler than you think to alter the state of resistance to learning. Here's an idea: learn one thing, practice it well, then use it as a launch pad to learn another thing well, then another and another.

Whether you see tai chi as a fighting method or an exercise, it's a *practice* at its core—a routine activity that you engage in, in order to improve and maintain specific kinds of movement for a multitude of results, such as overall health and longevity.

A true practice is incremental, steady, regular, and consistent over time. Even a little bit now and again adds up. The more you do the moves, the more you benefit. It helps to practice consistently with mindful attempts to recall what you were exposed to in class.

Tai chi is also a process of discovery. Each move that you learn is a stepping stone to learning more. More about how your body moves. More about how you think about moving. More about feeling the deeper components of movement and not just what you notice on the surface.

Perhaps our perfection resides in the notion that we desire to be better at what we do by simply trying. Unless we neglect our responsibility, we are assured success by virtue of our efforts. Desire transforms into intention; perception transforms into greater awareness. We perceive the obscure and it materializes into a tai chi practice.

What to Practice: Do the Basics and Build Momentum

My approach for a beginner and beyond is to do basic, fundamental moves. I write about these throughout *Practicing Tai Chi*. Everything you do builds upon the practice of the basics.

Most everyone practices form—linking postures with transitions from one to another. At first, most of us have trouble remembering the sequence steps and postures. But if you practice moves that you do remember, even the simplest ones, your body will feel the difference from trying. Then it will want more.

Many people have made tai chi a lifelong pursuit of skill and knowledge simply by employing universal, fundamental concepts and principles in everyday movements. Once you have a working understanding of the fundamentals, and then are incorporating them in your movements (not just tai chi), you can say you're doing tai chi— the "supreme, ultimate" expression of what you're doing at any moment.

So, I say learn the basics and learn them from a good teacher, someone who is passionate, humble, experienced, well-traveled, well-schooled, seeks simplicity, and teaches with kindness. Look for a teacher who is a good student, because only a good student can be a good teacher.

If It's Too Easy, Go Deeper

Even though you hear how easy the tai chi moves are, you might also hear that if it feels too easy, then you probably aren't aware of how much more deeply you could be doing it. I teach many things so learners can go deeper into more-detailed adjustments.

If you remember only the first few postures of the form, for example, it's enough to practice. Learn them with a clear purpose of going deeper into them. The posture shape, mind intention, focus of attention, drilling specific shapes, patterns and repetitions.

No one ever learns all there is to know and we are always learning. Remember that if it seems too easy, then you are not going deeply enough. A teacher should be able to help you go deeper because he or she has done so in mind, energy and body. A good teacher understands the energy. Few seem to study the more elusive, but richly rewarding, energetic dynamics of internal martial arts.

"You cannot change nature, only yourself."

Motivation and the No-Option Option

I'm interested in what motivates people to do tai chi in the first place and in what motivates them to continue practicing over the long term. What motivates them to begin may not be the same as what keeps them practicing for years. It could very well be, but I do believe that initial stimulus matures and evolves into something more. In fact, tai chi (and qigong, as well) can help you gather the will and energy to achieve life goals.

One important goal is to integrate some sort of "practice" in our daily lives that helps us to rise above external demands (often unwelcome), and integrate mind and body connectivity—in movement and thought—throughout the day. A practice can help to develop greater awareness of our deeper selves and awaken to that in the midst of life's daily challenges.

Our motivations are unique to each of us, but I believe that people go to their first tai chi class because they are seeking change. The specific change is unique to each of us. Once we do attend our first few classes, some of us have to consciously seek further motivation to continue. If we don't know how to proceed, we might not try. I say just do the moves. Learn them, remember them, do them.

Sometimes I think people correlate tai chi with "work." How could doing a few moves that feel good be work? We're so habituated to resisting "work," that we may be hindered from developing a beneficial exercise practice, or even from taking responsibility for our own health. Even if it does feel like work, this kind of "tai chi work" actually feels good. And that other work? Well, it drains you.

"It is better to do a single move perfectly than to do a hundred mediocre moves."
—old taiji saying—

Many of us have become complacent in our discomfort or mental fatigue. "Better the devil we know than the devil we don't know," as the saying goes. Well, that's not acceptable anymore when you give yourself over to learning something like tai chi. It was an enlightened moment when we took the initiative to try tai chi. Keep that in mind when you feel resistance.

Often, a distinct difference exists between the motivation that regular tai chi class participants feel in class and the lack of motivation at home. Getting motivated in class is easier than motivating yourself at home. At home you might begin a routine, but wear out before you reach a new level of attainment. If that comes up, just recall that moment that you first decided to give it a try. A nugget of motivation sprouts in that moment that will keep you going.

I think a lot of people discontinue tai chi practice because they think it would be too much of a full-time job learning tai chi. They're right. It is a full-time job for those who choose to make it one. It doesn't have to be so involved for everyone. You can do tai chi at whatever regularity that feels good. You can do more or you can do less.

What everyone should consider, however, is to put in enough time when you first begin learning in order to get the basics. What is not an option is to not to do tai chi at all.

I once read an article about a man sitting by a pond in an urban park who, while contemplating suicide with a gun hidden in his jacket, was approached by an elderly Chinese man who noticed him and asked if he was having a problem. He answered, "I can't sleep."

The Chinese man, who turned out to be the taiji master, T.T. Liang, said, "If I could show you how to sleep, would you be interested in learning?" The man said yes, so Master Liang taught him one move, the first move of the form, for 90 minutes.

The man was so tired and sore from what Master Liang showed him that he slept like a baby that night and forgot about killing himself. That was 50 years ago and he is still practicing and teaching others "how to sleep," as he says.

I tell this story to show that this man knew his motivation and you should know yours. It should be clear and sustainable, and should not falter. Never give up and see where it takes you. You see, for me taiji is more important than many other things in life. Period. Develop your private practice and see what I mean.

Even a little bit now and again adds up, but a true practice is incremental, steady, regular, and consistent over time.

Knowing Where and How to Begin is Key

I think many novices stumble at initiating a regular practice routine, not because they are not motivated; rather because they don't see how or where to begin. We might not have a motivation problem if we knew what to practice in the first place.

The beginning is probably the most difficult for learners. Serious tai chi is full of information and thresholds to pass through. However, you *are* rewarded for every sincere effort you make. And it takes less effort than you think. Of course, you won't know unless you try.

Knowing where to begin a practice session helps with shifting smoothly from regular daily activities to a tai chi routine. It doesn't matter what you practice so much, at least at first. My suggestion here is to see in your mind's eye an image of something you learned and let your feeling follow it, then do it with the body. Allow it to happen and it will.

In order for these steps to work, it would help to remember something that you learned from group class and can recall to begin a solo session. Just about anything is good for starting. I give you a lot of things in this book to tap into.

"Master yourself to master tai chi."

Be clear on where to begin in your practice. Standing in *wuji*, described later, is the most natural place to begin. Actually, it's "the" beginning! Then focus on something specific; for example, moving the sacrum or the dantian in specific shapes and patterns—circles, figure 8s, diagonals, spirals. I discuss these in following sections.

Trying to remember one thing can stimulate momentum. You can open the lower back (*ming men*): hip sink down, waist rise up, spine elongates, vertebrae open and separate, top of head rises, back of neck fills ("*xu ling ding jing*"). One of my teachers has called this (or something like it) "raising the *shen*." I call it a "one-minute exercise."

At first, emphasize actual physical parts of the body that need more movement. This is "structural." Later, if you practice regularly, you use this to further cultivate skill at visualizing and perceiving less corporeal things, such as *qi*. This can be potentially more powerful than moving just bones, joints, ligaments, tendons, and muscles. Ultimately, both of these "levels" complement each other when they align together in unity, synchronicity.

The truth is you're always at a starting point at which you're at a new learning edge. It's a chance to learn something you didn't know before. Sometimes that's uncomfortable. But if there's anything that we human beings are good at, it's overcoming the obstacle of not knowing something and learning anyway. You just have to trust.

I see trust as a letting go, but without loss of control. You're letting go of one kind of holding on to acquire a different kind of control based on accepting a basic *yin-yang* notion: although nothing can stay the same in a world of constant motion and change, a calm forms the center of that motion. Once you begin to perceive and grasp this, you begin to gain control.

Use Your Senses

I see tai chi as a tool to improve what we have already been doing: walk, stand, sit, breathe, see, feel, smell, hear, touch. It offers a way to improve how our senses function. Think of learning tai chi as a way of using your senses to learn. Our senses are our guides, even senses that are not so obvious, like heart feeling, or spirit-like revelations, or insights of the mind.

As the base senses sharpen, you will naturally taste differently and your sense of smell will heighten, your sense of touch will become more sensitive and alert, you vision may even improve. You will in-corporate these changes into your movement gradually, or maybe even in leaps and bounds. You will find your pace, and your tai chi legs will be increasingly able to manage bigger seas, so to speak.

Along with our senses, we were born with an inherent ability to change how we perceive—to adapt our conscious attention to see something in our actions that we had not noticed before. Perception exists in different forms: thought, feeling, emotion, sight, hearing, taste, touch, even movement. We perceive through movement itself. Perception is a motion of the view of one's surroundings.

Perception and awareness are at the root of taijiquan, or more pre-cisely, internal martial arts, or even more essentially—the *art of internal movement*.

When to Do Tai Chi: Timing

Lack of time is the number one reason why people don't practice. They don't have time because of greater demands. This is difficult to accept since tai chi for me is as necessary as eating and sleeping. One cool thing is that it replaces some exercise that we're not getting any-way.

Whether it's a daily practice or every other day, don't let it go too long before you do practice, because you will forget more than you wish. To facilitate memory, practice regularly with not too much time between practices.

Do tai chi just after returning home from class. Don't slip into old habits too quickly. Don't watch TV for a while. Practice one or two things you remember first.

Simplicity is essential. The simpler the better, because it facilitates remembering.

Practice a little when the urge comes to you of its own accord. Practice when your body calls for it. When you feel the urge, respond. Sooner or later, you will feel the urge. The most important time to do it is when you think of it during the course of the day. Do it when you think about doing it. Don't just continue to think about it, don't even talk about it—with yourself or anyone else. Just move with it.

Do tai chi especially when you are least likely to remember or don't feel like practicing. Trying to remember could help you through. Times of resistance are opportunities. In the past as a beginner, if I had remembered, I would have stopped to do a little tai chi.

The residual effect of the tai chi you did last week helps a little bit during such times. But you need to water yourself like you water your flowers.

How to Remember Better

Have you ever read something, then right after, you realize that you don't remember what it was you just read? Tai chi is like that, except it's not about reading. It's about doing movement. We take a class, we do all the moves, class ends, we leave the studio, we walk to our vehicles, go home, then forget what we had just done. So, when it occurs to us to practice at home, we don't know where to begin.

I recommend practicing after class at least one thing on your own to facilitate memory. This is a learning trick commonly employed in many other learning environments, such as with school subjects or learning a musical instrument. Take a few minutes to go over the material right after a class as a way to assimilate and internalize the information.

For many learners remembering the movements takes more effort than we expect it to because we forget right after doing them. You might realize at some point that learning tai chi requires a different kind of attention than we are accustomed to employing as we learn. What is the nature of that attention?

Some might refer to "body memory," but what is that overused phrase and do they know exactly what it is when they evoke it? One thing I know fairly clearly is that the body learns by doing, and by doing we build up a memory incrementally, one piece upon another, one experience upon another.

Some things are easier to remember when they're simple to do. The caveat is if it is too simple the learner may lose interest. There must also be a challenge. But no matter what, you must seek to focus on remembering something that resonates in order to receive the benefits.

With practice, you'll recall newly introduced things more quickly. Fortunately, the benefits are cumulative. Our bodies store the information indefinitely. Many people start and stop practice, then if and when they start back up, they think they forgot everything and will have to start from scratch. But even after not practicing for a while, you pick it right back up again. Your body remembers and it's like you're right back where you left off like it was yesterday.

Group and Solo Practice and Social Connection

My experience as a student and teacher has taught me that practicing in a group setting at least twice a week, along with some solo practice at home, works well for learning and remembering.

Working regularly with others stimulates learning. It stimulates skill building, too, as well as a chance to overcome forgetfulness. At first, class is to learn the basics, but you can also use it to gauge progress in home practice. Focus on remembering one thing that stands out. Bring it home and practice it. Test your solo-practice outcomes in class with others. Your learning will skyrocket.

I strongly recommend a weekend workshop at least once a year. What you learn in tai chi class accumulates into a mass of information, little of which you may be clear about unless you practice sufficiently with others for a longer period of time than an occasional class.

My teacher told us learners in an all-day practice: "If you want to make the world a better place, then make yourself a better person."

Tai chi practice engages us in social connection. It can orient us to the external world and even help shape our worldview. To change the body and to assume a posture in such a way in order to accomplish a certain result often evokes a big change of mind and our feelings and presumptions about ourselves. My teacher told us learners in an all-day practice: "If you want to make the world a better place, then make yourself a better person."

A practitioner can work with others and act honorably and honestly with compassion and wisdom. Not an easy thing to do in a society in which self-gratification is such a powerful force; so much so, that it affects us all, thus making it difficult to hold to a course of self-improvement.

Tai chi practice is actually a way of creating intention for the purpose of cultivating self-awareness that allows us to act in ways that are often difficult to do in the day-to-day world. It's a way to remove ourselves from worldly indulgences for a little while so that we may practice being in the same state of mind that we cultivate in our practice.

And we don't have to do it alone, we can share it with other like-minded practitioners.

The Opponent

Most people do tai chi for health, not to fight. But the idea of an opponent can help a tai-chi-for-health practice, all the same. Your weaknesses are your opponents: faults, fears, injuries, chronic conditions, and so on. Those thoughts and feelings and actions that you perhaps wouldn't even tell your best friend about. Only you know. You live with them and they reside in memories, many you wish had never come to be and would forget if you could.

The concept of an opponent relates to the motivation to do tai chi in the first place, which is to either prevent or overcome some challenge. By virtue of this dynamic we have an opponent that must be overcome in order to succeed in our quest—our practice. To achieve the goals of practice is to overcome an opponent.

The adversary is obvious for some and maybe tai chi can help with quality-of-life management. Parkinson's, multiple sclerosis, and other autoimmune diseases. Arthritis, diabetes, depression, anxiety. Sometimes the adversary is less clear, but no less ominous: aging, dementia, Alzheimer's, chronic fatigue syndrome, fibromyalgia, ADHD, PTSD. We have acute injuries to heal, digestive issues to solve, and so on.

These opponents are not standing in front of you with a weapon aiming to annihilate you. They lurk below the surface constantly stalking you, wearing on your body and your resolve. You can't fight back like you may be able to against someone facing you. It's not a battle that you fight, then it's over. We don't even know what these adversaries are. Little seems to throw light on their true nature.

Ultimately, even with all the resources we have in medical care, we find ourselves alone with our opponent. Our only resource is our own will power and a practice. Maybe we don't completely overcome these opponents, but we can overcome our inaction towards them by developing a practice of simple concentration and meditative movement.

CHAPTER FOUR

Activities and Concepts for Tai Chi Practice

This is a good guide for doing tai chi: Even when you're wrong, you're right. For beginners, there is only where you are in your learning and what you are doing to progress.

You can Google "how to do tai chi" and get as many as 1.9 million results (when I looked). But what are you actually doing when you do tai chi and qigong?

For me as a learner and instructor, tai chi is made up of categories of exercise activities: visualization, breathing meditation, loosening, stretching, energy cultivation, form practice, standing and sitting meditation, single-basic repetitions, walking drills, two-person practice and testing, or sensitivity training.

I describe these activities for doing tai chi, as well as *concepts* to immerse more into the study of tai chi. Each activity describes a milestone in learning that can mark your progress in building skill and knowledge.

Not all the concepts that I describe are easy to grasp, especially just from reading about them. You have to do them with someone who knows how. My teachers emphasize them and I teach them in my *Fundamentals* course. They can also form the bulk of a home practice.

The Six Directions

In its simplest form, tai chi can be understood as movement in six directions and a few shapes and patterns of movement. The six directions are up/down, front/back, left/right. Every move you make incorporates one at a time or all at the same time. You can focus your attention on one at a time at first as a practice method.

Here are two things to remember about the six directions. When you move up, you move down at the same time. One produces the other. This is the *Yin-Yang* principle. It is not just up or just down, it's both simultaneously or in succession. Same for front-back and left-right. My teacher calls this "opposing forces," but I like to describe it as "dynamic tension." It's like pushing and pulling at the same time.

Keep in mind also that when you are moving all six directions simultaneously you will be spiraling. This is the very essence of movement in tai chi and other Chinese internal martial arts.

In tai chi class, we practice with awareness of intentionally moving in the six directions. This should help to cultivate a greater sense of balance and to recognize where our "central equilibrium" is—the center line, or plumb line, from the top of head to the ground between the ankles. I encourage everyone to "move around it," not just "move it around." Move up and down its length. Forward and back. Left and right. Straight, strong, alive, flexible, always regenerating.

Visualization

Incorporate visualization—picturing movement in order to facilitate learning. This is a crucial ingredient to make learning a more-effective and powerful process. Perceiving a different way of moving than the one we're use to is one of the benefits of visualizing. One trick I use is to simply go through the moves of a form in my mind. I picture each move as it follows the previous one. This mental practice helps to recall new things more readily. You also cultivate greater skill at visualizing itself.

Becoming Aware (Meditation)

As I've said before, tai chi is a form of meditation in which you move your body with a mindful intention to the manner in which you're moving. This approach to meditation and movement produces obvious positive results in a number of areas, including improved balance and blood circulation, particularly to the brain, and an overall sense of well-being and more energy. Explanations of this phenomena fall short of how and why these results take place. Indeed, researchers in science fields are really only recently turning more rigorous attention to the subject.

Reminder:
We learn tai chi by doing tai chi. Do the moves!

When you're doing tai chi, you're cultivating awareness of a multitude of things, but when you begin you need only to focus your attention on one or two things at a time. One is what your body is feeling. For example, be attentive to the feeling of the soles of the feet on the ground or floor. Is your jaw tight, lips pressed, mouth open? Do your ears feel plugged? Which muscles are tight? What is your breathing like?

Throughout your practice you will probably always be seeking to be aware of tension, or "clenching" and "torqued" parts of your body. And your intention will be to release it. You will in time if you keep in mind that tai chi movement itself is the way to relax the stress points. It's a gradual process of coaxing your body and your mind to cooperate to move smoothly with a flowing, effortless motion. The movement helps you loosen, relax and release.

Practice builds up the ability to hold in awareness many things simultaneously. There is a special dynamic between body and mind in which you can change the mind to change the body, but until you move the body, the mind may not cultivate an awareness of what to do. It's continual feedback between the parts: the mind, energy, body.

Visualization is the first step in picturing movement, but you can go further.

See, Feel, Do

Reading a book about how to do tai chi is not the same as learning by doing. And while learning by reading helps to develop one's mental picture, the body still has to do it to learn. Your body does not "read," at least not the way we normally think of it. It requires a different kind of text—the text of seeing, feeling and doing.

Training your attention is key
to all activity in tai chi and qigong.

The masters say the progression of movement should be mind, energy, physical (or *yi-qi-li*). I tell my students to "see, feel, do." You can develop greater sensitivity to subtle energies and changes in the six directions by practicing this mind-energy-body progression of movement.

The simplest way I know to practice effectively is to patiently visualize a move before actually moving. More precisely, I simply focus my attention on the point from where I want to initiate movement. When I do that, *qi* goes there in a natural response to the intention that's been set. As a result of this, the body follows, completing the three-phase progression of see, feel, do.

This is a powerful way to focus your attention in meditative movement. The significance of this, and the challenge, too, is understated by its simplicity. You might find that it can be deceptive when you actually try to do it. You might find that you're trying to break a fixation held by habituated movement.

Focusing on a single point single-mindedly is a stepping stone in the practice of tai chi. Every phase of your journey is performed by using this method of attention gathering. It is a technique for becoming familiar with the concept of tai chi movement and waking up to the possibility of moving differently from what you're used to.

With that, you learn something about moving in general. More significantly, you learn about attention itself and how powerful it can be to shift it from stagnant, fixated views to even an inkling of an alternative. Your task, is to cultivate the ability to do that.

I have often heard Master Xu refer to focusing on specific places and activities. He's probably talking about more than what his words signify to most of his listeners. He repeats himself so many times in his discussions that the repetition draws attention to itself. So, for a serious practitioner of internal martial arts, "see, feel, do" must be understood as an important key to successful growth.

Rationale

The nature of movement stems from mind wanting or desiring. When we were infants we could not move our bodies, but we could see. We learned about the world, our surroundings, only through seeing, and feeling as well, but we could not, for some time, reach out and touch the world. We could only want to.

Over time as we grew up, we downplayed this progression of seeing, feeling, then doing and replaced it with doing, all doing, no attention to seeing or feeling, which are taken for granted. But, they're still crucial parts of our being. Indeed, they existed before the doing and made the doing possible in the first place. We just lost touch with the progression of see, feel, do.

Standing in *Wuji*

Wuji is the first position in the form, where you begin before doing anything else in tai chi. One way to begin is to find your *zhong ding*, your up-down centerline, or your "central equilibrium." Physically, your ears are over the shoulders, which are in line with the hips, which are in line with the knees and ankles and the "Bubbling

Spring" (*Yongquan*)—the point behind the ball of the foot and to the center.

You will probably have to slightly bend and/or "soften" the knees to get there, maybe tilt the pelvis one way or another. This physical alignment is only part of *wuji*. It's a place to begin to train your attention.

Even when you're moving, be in *wuji*, that still center. Within that stillness, there is aliveness. There is no movement without stillness and no stillness without movement.

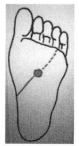

Bubbling Spring

Every time you stand in *wuji* you are beginning again, perhaps a little farther along than the last time you practiced.

> *Stand in Wuji: Sincere and patient, but not neglectful.*
> *Stand in Wuji: Stable and rooted, yet agile and poised.*
> *Stand in Wuji: Sky comes down to you, Earth rises up.*
> *Stand in Wuji: Even in movement, the stillness is Yin, the conscious center.*

Breath and Breathing

Breath and breathing are important in tai chi. For a while in classes, I did not talk about the role of breathing. Internal martial arts teachers I've studied with say not to focus on breathing. "Breathe naturally," they would say. They never explained why, but I suspect they concluded that my fellow learners and I were not ready to hear about the subtler aspects of breath and breathing in martial arts. We were there for different things. Either that, or breathing just was not important for them.

However, many beginning tai chi learners don't have a practice of controlled breathing, which is a clear sign that they are hindered from relaxing and developing greater skill.

Part of the stress syndrome is a poor breathing habit. So now, along with many other things that I discuss with learners, studied breathing offers an entryway into practicing tai chi. I offer pointers on consciously including breathing techniques applicable in both sitting and moving meditation.

There is so much information (Cohen, 1997; Jou, 1997) about breathing benefits and techniques that it's nearly pointless to talk about it here. But I still have something to say about it from my perspective as an instructor and practitioner.

There's more to it than meets the eye, and breathing is only the beginning into seeing more about the possibilities of any given movement in qigong or tai chi—or any kind of movement for that matter. Breathing is huge whether you do tai chi or not. You can never overestimate the power of breath and breathing. Breath is the thread of life, a magical lifeline.

Both qigong and tai chi breathing are similar to sitting meditations, but differ because you incorporate movement with them. Plus, different breaths can be utilized for various purposes.

In sitting meditation, breathing is a main focus while you silence the mind. This kind of focused breathing practice produces many various effects in the body and mind, even the emotions. It can affect both your sympathetic and parasympathetic nervous systems.

During moving meditation, I bring attention to breath only at specific times. The majority of practice is natural breathing which my teacher and others sometimes referred to as "subconscious" breathing. We simply don't notice, or pay attention to, our breathing in this case. It's natural.

One of the times in which breath plays a role in movement is simply to begin a move or complete a move. Sometimes, it helps to focus on adding an inhalation or exhalation to finish. It helps to give shape to the body while executing a movement.

I suggest practicing breathing technique while sitting or walking at times other than when doing tai chi or qigong. Practice just breathing. With mindful attention to your breathing technique you can induce relaxation, better posture, circulation, concentration. You can decrease stress, muscle and joint tension, chronic pain and much more. It doesn't matter who you are; you need to breathe better.

One of the times in which breath plays a role in movement is simply to begin or complete a move.

Most, if not all, teachers of meditation and qigong encourage learners first to develop proficiency at breathing abdominally. Abdominal breathing is a method to help teach the body to open the ribs and upper chest laterally, adding more oxygen to the lower part of the lungs, fill the back of the neck and the lower back/kidney area with breath, lower the center of gravity, keep the shoulders down and generate a slow, relaxing beta frequency, all the while providing more oxygen to the blood and ultimately to the brain, organs and cells.

Note that keeping shoulders down is not a final goal, but a sign of whether or not you're doing the more beneficial postural action. You're not if your shoulders rise and tense up. However, if your shoulders don't come up while you move doesn't necessarily mean you are correct. You may be forcing it rather than letting it sink freely and rest on the waist and hips. But chances are that you may be correct and you're on the path.

The position of the upper and lower body is a key factor in the breath's ability to fill the lungs. Posture is also key to the ability to execute a movement fully and having power with it.

I'm always amazed at how differently focused, controlled breathing helps us to feel and to move. Whether you're sitting still or moving, develop a breathing practice and see it change how you feel.

Other modes of breath control are reverse breathing and whole-body breathing, or absorbing breath, which I believe is also called turtle breathing and skin breathing (see Jou, Tsung Hwa, 1983, for his discussions on breathing).

Limits of Breath in Tai Chi

To reiterate, while important in many aspects and practices, breath is not always a leading, determining factor in the effectiveness of a practice. Mind intention (*Shen*) directing *qi* is characteristic of a more mature phase of learning.

Through my own explorations, I've come to believe that too much focus on breath in movement limits what you are able to do with energy and mind intention. Breath, especially for beginners and intermediates, can be used to help guide *qi*, but further on, mind intention directs *qi* to a part of the body, and even beyond, for specific actions to occur.

You can also place single-minded attention on *qi* (life force) and its movement. *Qi* can extend beyond the body. Mind intention directs it. You simply have to practice the moves and the principles, and discover this.

The message here is: don't let breath be the only focus of your attention when doing tai chi moves. Keep in mind that breath is part of a greater context in which *Shen* and *Qi* play a more extensive role.

Breathing Exercises

Find out what kind of breather you are

Take a deep breath while resting a hand on your chest and the other on your stomach. If your chest inflates and your shoulders rise, but there is no expansion in your torso, you're a chest breather. Most (untrained) adults breathe like this.

More beneficial breathing entails expanding your torso 360 degrees. The most obvious change is the belly expanding outward on the inhale and contracting (relaxing) on the exhale. The lower back expands as well as the abdomen. I find it relaxing to breathe this way. Pressure is reduced on the sciatic muscles.

Babies, cats and dogs are really good examples of this kind of breathing. Relaxed, full and complete.

Breathing Exercise #1—Dantian Awareness Breathing

Place the tip of your index finger on the navel with the other fingers lined up below it. Roll you fingers and press inward where your pinky finger is. That's just about where it is said the *dantian* is located—about two inches down and one-three inches in. For me, that's only a place to begin. Breathe into where your fingers are with small, brief bursts. Contain the up and down movement there only if possible. It takes concentration at first for many people to get the breathing to move just that spot.

Breathing Exercise #2—Relaxation Breathing

Lie down on your back with a chair facing you. Place your calves over the chair's seat. The calves are parallel to the floor and your thighs are perpendicular to it. Do breathing exercise #1 in this position.

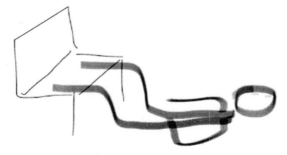

Breathing Exercise #3—Breathe Slowly, Steadily, Deeply

While standing in *wuji*, breathe really deeply into the abdomen so fully you can't inhale anymore air. The ribs expand, the belly expands. It even feels like your feet are pressing into the ground.

Relax when you exhale, not push it out forcefully, at least until you reach the end of the exhale. Then when out of air you push out the last residue of air from your lungs. Feels like your cells are squeezing toxins out of your skin much like squeezing the last drops of water from a dishtowel.

Note: Don't let shoulders lift, rather expand the ribs outward to sides, allowing shoulders to sit on waist and hip.

Caution: Stop and rest if you get light-headed or dizzy.

Be sure to breathe into the abdomen and let it fill everywhere from there; lungs as ribs expand, finger tips, toes, kidneys. Don't over extend, or force the movement. Intend the life regenerating breath with its oxygen and the nutrients it carries to the cells needed to grow and function optimally.

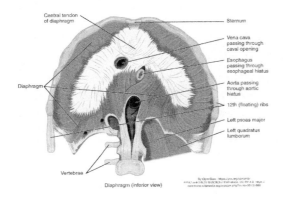

The Diaphragm

Breathing Exercise #4—Diaphragmatic Movement

Slightly different from abdominal breathing is to focus on the motion of the diaphragm to practice *diaphragmatic breathing*. To do it, flex the diaphragm up and down to change its shape from flat to a mushroom shape, then back and so on. This is intentional physical movement of the diaphragm independently as opposed to using breath alone to move. This method can be more efficient than abdominal breathing, especially while in motion, such as tai chi walking. Operatic singers know this action well.

Breathing Exercise #5—Visualize Breathing

Visualize the inhale and exhale through various locations in the body. For example, as the body moves, imagine inhaling and exhaling through the lower back as though through nostrils. Breathe into and out of the joints, the solar plexus, the soles of the feet and top of the head, the back of the neck. See how it changes how your body moves. The central equilibrium, gravity, *dantian*, open-close, left-right, front-back, left-right, big-little.

Appreciate the empty spaces within your being. Move from emptiness, return to emptiness.

This is a more meditative practice similarly described later in the small cosmic circuit practice. You don't have to practice tai chi to try this. Anyone can incorporate this simple tai chi breathing technique anytime during the day either sitting in meditation or walking. It relaxes and teaches the body and mind, plus it improves circulation, getting life-giving oxygen and nutrients into the blood stream.

Ways to Correct Your Breathing Form

Don't hold your breath if you are inclined to do that out of unexamined habit, stress, fear, uncertainty. Let it move freely, smoothly. Be mindful, focus your attention closely on your intent and the subtle changes that you can find in the movements. Perfecting and internalizing breathing form takes repeated attempts, so practice, practice, practice.

In qigong and tai chi, especially if you are a beginner, you can get good results by coordinating breath with movement. For example, you can inhale or exhale while your arms expand out or draw in as you time the speed of the movement to match the speed of inhale and exhale. Coordinating inhale and exhale with various arm movements: up-down, front-back, left-right can be a meditation.

Coordinating breath with movement can be part of tai chi and qigong learning, but doesn't need to be a central focus all the time. Mind and *qi* can be coordinated, as well, and should be a major focus of tai chi practice. This goes beyond breath.

Maybe you can do it in a qigong or tai chi class, but can you be aware of breath and motion while doing everyday things?

Qigong (氣功)

> *Focusing on external sight can remove heat Fire, while focusing on internal sight can warm Yang. Imagining a scene of Water and coldness can supplement Yin, while a mental-visualizing a scene of Fire and heat can elevate Yang*
>
> (Liu, Chinese Medical Qigong, 2013, p48).

Breath is a key component of *qigong*, or "energy work," or energy cultivation. Essentially, *qigong* is a practice of regulating breath, body and spirit, but you can find many definitions and explanations to boggle your mind. You can find many references to medical *qigong*, martial *qigong*, scholarly *qigong*, and *qigong* of a religious kind, such as in Taoism (see Yang, 1997; Cohen, 1997).

You will see different kinds of movements depending on whether you're doing tai chi or qigong, but at their core, energy, *qi*, or life force, is fundamental.

Qigong practice is as old as China, much older than taijiquan. But qigong relates to tai chi in that you can merge it into a movement awareness, by moving energy to move your body in tai chi postures and transitions.

Words can only approximate a description. It has to be felt. You may be able to see it or at least know what you are seeing as a result of it being present and active in the body and movement of someone doing tai chi.

With beginners, I practice what my teacher George Xu calls *Hun Yuan Qigong*—primordial energy cultivation. This qigong presumably comes from Grandmaster Feng Zhi Qiang (with whom Master Xu studied). It is part of the Chen style of *taijiquan*, for which Master Xu is known. You can look into it for your own study. I also follow qigong sets I've learned from a few other teachers, also from martial traditions.

Shen (神)

Often translated in *taijiquan* vernacular as mind intention, *shen* can also mean "spirit." Mind intention is a key component in movement that relates strongly to visualization practices. Employing *shen* by simply focusing the attention on a specific locus and task can be a major stepping stone in the learning tai chi. When you use mental visualization, you're making good use of your ability to perceive and to be more aware.

Zhong Ding and Dantian

Master practitioners of tai chi will tell you that *zhong ding* and *dantian* are two most important concepts in tai chi and Chinese internal martial arts. They are also the most basic. You will work on these two concepts for as long as you do tai chi. Hopefully, that will be a lifetime. It shouldn't take long to understand the concepts, but you can spend your life developing them for the profound benefits they offer.

Awareness of *zhong ding* and *dantian* in movement is a point of departure to begin cultivating movement awareness in two zones: externally and internally. External is awareness of the superficial movement as it is seen from the outside: the shape of the move, the speed; for example, the coordination of arms, waist, hips, and legs. I refer to these components as "structure," or the physical.

A little more internally, you focus on the movement of bones, joints, ligaments, tendons, even skin (or fascia) on one level. More deeply, internal is awareness of *qi* (energy) and *shen* (mind intention or intent). This is more abstract in quality and referred to as the "energetic," or "internal."

Zhong Ding

If you want to learn tai chi, you should know about *zhong ding*, or central equilibrium. *Zhong ding* work, or "gong" (along with its complement, *dantian gong*), is necessary to truly understand and enhance your practice of tai chi and qigong. Whether you practice for martial arts or longevity exercises, both are essential to make practice most effective. I could talk about it, explain it, define it and try to make sense of it in a book or blog post, but it is always better to just do it and learn through doing.

"Adjusting the mind also involves changes of Yin-Yang. Keeping the mind in focus and mental-visualization practice especially are fully characterized by variations of Yin and Yang.

Zhong ding as a key concept of tai chi and internal martial arts is just about the first thing I teach beginning tai chi learners. I particularly like introducing the concept for improving posture and stability. With greater awareness and skill, you can also move with more "power." I emphasize health and well-being, but martial application is well-within that range.

Zhong ding is especially important for emphasizing the internal focus of martial arts. Dedicated practitioners employ *zhong ding*, as well as *dantian*, to evolve greater ability and clarity in practice from the *inside out*.

You can employ *zhong ding* in countless ways in daily living, such as walking—a most natural activity. When I first discovered *zhong ding*—

meaning when I really felt it—I was walking in a forest of Ponderosa pine. The powerful presence of the tall, straight trunks must have attracted my subconscious and I suddenly felt my own spine align with them and lift up, almost in lockstep with them as I sauntered among them. It was a waking moment.

Dantian

Often, we start with the *dantian*: that point below the navel and inward a couple of inches. Instructors will say to move the waist. The instruction to "move the waist" simplifies much about tai chi movement, which usually takes beginners some repeated effort to become familiar and comfortable with.

The *dantian* is also thought of as a larger area with the point more or less in its center. The *dantian* is not just a place, but also a mental picture—a concept that you can formulate and locate anywhere. Doing tai chi can be a practice of placing this picture anywhere. You move with this idea in mind.

You can focus on three key *dantians*: the lower *dantian*, just described, the middle *dantian*, or solar plexus area, and the upper *dantian*, or the "mind's eye," or "third eye," an opening in the middle of the forehead between the eye brows.

Dantian = *Field of elixir, where life force is stored. It is where the* Jing *(essence) is converted to* Qi *(vital energy).* Jing *is the creative potential, sexual essence. Once the sperm unites with the egg, life begins to form.* Qi *is the energy of life and it is stored in the* Dantian.

A little story

In 2004, I asked Xu Guo Chang in Shanghai a question about *dantian* and he said not to worry about *dantian*. He said that for him everywhere is *dantian*. I've heard others ask similar questions and get similar answers. It sometimes seems as though a person is trying show off what they know when they ask such a question, when in fact they actually know very little.

In my case, I needed a place to anchor my learning. A place to begin. That was my first trip to China and I was aware that I knew very little. But I needed to ask something to engage the teacher—anything from which to build.

I know more now and I understand what is meant by "everywhere is *dantian*." At least what I think it is. It works for me in my practice. Until I learn something new or different, this is a working definition that I can apply in practice.

Both, *dantian* and *zhong ding*, apply to more than fighting technique, but to everyday life. The ability to move is magical and how we move has potential to change how the external environment reacts to our presence. Many people are suffering needlessly, in my view, when all they could do is to learn to move differently, with intention and clarity, and demonstrate awareness and ability.

Ways to Practice Feeling & Moving the Dantian

You can focus on moving both physically and energetically in tai chi practice. You can move the *dantian* with a focus on both, either separately or simultaneously. I practice three ways of moving the *dantian* that primarily incorporate the physical and energetic.

One…Qi Circles

I lead groups in a variety of single-basic movement sets to practice circles. I learned them from my Chen style practice with Master Xu (Richard, 18 Circles), and Susan A. Matthews, but also Wu style practice with Grandmaster Wang Hao Da (see Richard, "Wang Hao Da Neijing Training" in References).

Circles can be both physical and energy movement. To practice, visualize a circle in your abdomen and move your mental attention around the perimeter of the circle as though it were a ball or the crest of a wave—whatever appeals to you. This taps into the "area" concept of movement shape (see below). You can also see the activity as though the *dantian* point is the hub of a wheel and the movement is of the wheel turning around its hub.

Figure Eights

Combine two circles to make a figure eight and move within that shape. One circle is clockwise, the other counter-clockwise. Do this in waist and hips. You may have to train yourself to focus and concentrate in order to do it.

Why Qi Circles Are Important ...

...because they form the basis for more-refined movement, more conscious and aware of subtle flow of energy in and out of the body. More integrated mind/body and eventually spirit, with enough practice. In which the physical and energetic merge into more of a single consciousness ... to unify and become one. Rather than two, each with its own mind, you have one mind with two complementary parts—*Yin* and *Yang*.

Two...Change the Shape of the Dantian

Elongating the *dantian* into an oval shape is an easy enough thing to do. When you stretch up-down, opening the front of the body, your abdomen, stomach, ribs, etc. all squeeze inward in the front-back plane and upward and downward in the up-down plane. Sort of like you do when lifting weights, but with less tightening.

Three...Point to Ball, Shrink and Expand

This is described elsewhere, too. It wakes you up to the feeling of energy movement. Stand in *wuji* and hold your arms out in front of you as though holding a ball or wrapping them around a tree. Visualize a point just below the navel and inside your body a couple of inches. Don't think about breath. Simply visualize that point become a ball and then shrink back to a point. Repeat just visualizing. You don't have to open and close your arms, but it might feel natural to do so.

This exercise is designed to help you feel *qi*. Really, to help you feel, period.

Alignment, Area, and Volume

With a basic grasp of *zhong ding* and *dantian* in movement, you have enough to build upon to be familiar, comfortable and to refine your practice of tai chi movement (see page 27). My teacher, Xu Guo Ming (George), has characterized the "shape" and movement of energy regarding *zhong ding* and *dantian* in three ways: linear, area (circumference), and volume. Energy moves in shapes. This is a key concept to remember as you learn.

I include this information because I think it's good for keeping in mind as you progress in your learning and as you become more familiar with concepts and practices. This section will be available to you to review one future day.

Alignment

Alignment has a linear quality that we can become aware of in our bodies. I see its locus as a threadlike center line from the crown of the head through the middle of the body lengthwise down to the ground between the *bubbling springs* of each foot. It runs just in front of the spine. With practice and familiarity, you can see or feel it also winding through the marrow of the bones, present in every fraction of the length of the body. It is dynamic, alive, in motion, adjusting and renewing itself continually. It has an up-down quality to it.

The shortest distance between two points is a straight line. Moving between those two points requires the least amount of effort. Tai chi is all about producing maximum results from minimum effort, so alignment is one practice you can develop.

For example, if you hold your gaze on the *bubbling spring* and the *dantian* simultaneously and practice perceiving movement up and down between the two, you will develop a "two-point correspondence" between them. Through movement, the parts—*bubbling spring, dantian,* and space between them—become a single unit. They move in harmony.

This can also bring the concept of "opposing forces" into perspective. This term I think is meant to be opposite forces, meaning up/down simultaneously, not two forces colliding or going against each other.

Actually, you never want to "go against." In tai chi, you must "yield" and redirect the force from an opponent. Rather, use up-down to open, separate, and extend the line between the two points (to and from one to the other continually, simultaneously) to redirect the opposing force.

Area and Volume

Along with alignment, we use area and volume to balance ourselves in response to the pressures from outside. Almost everything we do is a response to some pressure from some external force in our environment. The environment could be the physical environment near us or it could be a more abstract environment—distant and foreign.

I've learned that central equilibrium is more than alignment. Equilibrium, which we can become aware of and utilize in movement, is alignment in relation to our environment, but it's more multi-dimensional. It has area and volume, not just up/down linearly.

Area is the edge, the line around the perimeter of our energetic shape. You can move in circles with attention to this idea of a line that draws a circumference around you. I do this when doing *qi* circles in vertical, horizontal and diagonal planes.

Volume extends in all directions and fills up with awareness and *qi*. It is front/back and left/right, as well as up-down. It is a point that expands into a sphere, or a ball, in our perception. You can visualize this in practice and you can feel it. You can direct it and other people can feel you doing it, too. The *dantian* has a lot to do with volume.

Whole Body Moves as a Single Unit

You move through phases of practice during which you come to understand a number of concepts that you incorporate back into practice. "Whole body moves as a single unit" is one and it's one of the first concepts I work with learners to understand. It's a major milestone to reach in your understanding. The old teachers often refer to this as "harmony." You could think of it also as "synchrony." The *dantian* and *zhong ding* work in unison to produce whole body movement. The first thing to become aware of is whether you're "connected" or not. This means essentially that if one part of the body moves, then all the rest move with it. If one part is not moving, then none should be.

> *"This marvel must be grasped intuitively and cannot be expressed in words. Only when it is known in the mind can the body know it; but knowing with the body is superior to knowing with the mind."*
>
> *("Taijiquan Treatise" in Wile, D.,*
> *Lost T'ai Chi Classics from the Late Ch'ing Dynasty.)*

Usually, we rely on individual parts as surrogates for moving the whole body. Often, when we bend over to retrieve a fallen spoon or something that slips from your hands to the ground, we can't quite reach it, so we extend the arm out more to reach it. This is what is called "breaking," or stretching whatever you can while other parts of the body hold back. You can throw your back out, or at least feel strain.

Learning to move as a single unit really helps to alleviate this poor practice. Instead we could try positioning the body to take advantage of employing all the bones, joints, ligaments and tendons in unison. Breath, too. This would reduce pressure placed on any single part.

One way to approach understanding this is, is to cultivate awareness of two things: parts of your body that are moving and parts that are not moving. It's the parts you're not moving that can hinder your ability to be in equilibrium and move smoothly and fully.

It takes practice, not because it's a difficult concept, but rather, people are so out of balance and move so incoherently that we have to get through a lot to open our minds to the concept of "unit."

I find that to learn unit, beginners and intermediate practitioners do fairly well by learning to initiate a move from one locus in the body, get more or less proficient at it, then shift their focus to another place and move from there. This relates to the concepts of see, feel, do. It also relates to the traditional idea of a "string of pearls"—each joint is like a pearl and the energy that connects them is the string. It's a continuous, unbroken chain through which energy, thus the body, moves.

I often begin with the *bubbling spring*, but just as often with the *dantian*. You initiate movement, then try to feel how the impulse of energy can travel through the rest of the body. Eventually, you are able to hold the image of more and more points of movement, until they appear to move synchronously—all the parts contributing to the whole.

To reiterate a recurring theme in this book: focus your attention on one point and/or activity and sustain that concentration during movement.

"Unit" Practice Points

How would you know you're moving the whole body as a single unit? Most people don't feel many, if not most, parts moving. Cultivating an awareness of this is the function of tai chi movement. So, where do you begin? In the beginning, the focus of your attention would be on choosing an activity to begin. For example, moving the arms in harmony with breath. Here's a way to do that.

Inhale (or exhale) and raise the arms to each side shoulder height and parallel to the floor or ground (a T shape). Time the move so that the breath initiates the move and ends at the same time the movement ends. Changing direction, exhale and drop arms to the side with the same coordinated timing. Pretty simple, huh? Do the same thing again, this time raise the arms in front of you as in the first move of the form.

This activity is good for novices because of its simplicity. It is limited, however, because it's focusing only on a section of the body, not the body as a whole. But it does give you a chance to practice coordinating breath with movement of the body, and even help to establish an awareness of how you can coordinate moving *qi* and the body together in harmony.

Keep in mind that the difference is in focusing on a specific activity initiated from a specific locus, the rest of the body settles into harmony—the motion of the parts become the sum of the whole in motion (see visualizing expand/shrink dantian, point/ball exercise). Kind of interesting, plus it feels pretty good when you recognize it's happening.

Weighted in Gravity

"Gravity" is another milestone and an important concept in tai chi practice. Relaxed and sunk is way of describing it. The Chinese term, *Fang Sung,* is a related concept. In gravity, you're not lifting with muscle. Everything—bones, joints, ligaments, tendons, skin—rests like a stone on the ground, or water seeking the lowest level. A feather drifting downward. Coins stacked one upon the other. Not lifting up, not tensing up or clenching. Not pushing downward either, just there, heavy, unaffected. Not dead, but dead-like. What moves the body is mind (*yi*) intention, (*shen*) and *qi*.

Try this: Stand in *wuji* and focus on your sacrum. Focus on feeling spine, sacrum, tailbone in alignment with the bubbling well. Visualize a dropping of the whole spine. This "letting go" is not from bending joints, but a feeling of deep, inner release. It's like the body lets out a big sigh, but does not collapse. You feel "gravity": the weight of your arms and shoulders is obvious. The shoulder joints, hip, spine feel heavy. Muscle lets go. Joints also "open" and "expand," filling with space and, presumably, *qi*.

Gravity Exercise

You and a partner stand side-by-side and you raise your arm and let it rest in your partner's hand. Just let it drop without holding it up. Let the other person hold it up. This should give you an initial idea of weighted in gravity. You can develop an ability to feel the whole body do the same heavy falling feeling.

Zhan Zhuang—Standing

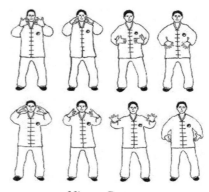

Yiquan Postures

Standing, or *Zhan Zhuang*, is the practice of holding a posture for an extended period of time. A couple of minutes at a time is enough for a beginner. The secret to standing in *zhan zhuang* (or *yi quan*, which is similar) is not in how still you can be, rather how you adapt and adjust subtle energies in the body so that you will be relaxed, yet strong, calm, yet alert.

Trying not to move can create tension and defeat the purpose of standing. Start with observing breath, muscles and positions of the joints. Look for where you feel tense or out of alignment. Energy must fill and flow freely. If not, then you are holding on to something that hinders flow.

You can incorporate standing principles when you pause in a posture in the form; then maintain the sense, or sensation cultivated in standing, as you move through transitions from one posture to another.

This is very similar to wuji and maintaining a still center while in the midst of movement.

Awareness of alignment—i.e., central equilibrium/*zhong ding*—and *Qi* flowing and circulating through everything is the essence of tai chi. This is "stillness in movement." *Wuji* never goes away even though you are moving. Very *Yin-Yang*.

You can learn more about standing by reading *The Way of Energy* by Lam, Kam-Chuen. I think it's a decent introduction for beginners or practitioners looking for more insight. Master Lam has produced many free youtube.com video lessons, as well.

Loosening

I believe that you should do loosening movements before you do stretching postures. Loosening joints, ligaments, tendons, muscles is key to a well-rounded practice. I incorporate loosening in single-basic repetitions.

Maybe I could describe how to loosen in a book somehow, but it would not be anywhere close to doing it with someone who is familiar with it. So, here, I just refer to it so you will know about it and perhaps find a way to learn more. I'm always available to help in my classes, of course.

Many students of tai chi don't move the hips enough or not at all. Usually, they are not aware of this. Loose, open hips can help alleviate knee problems and low back pain. There are moves, postures, stances, and mind intention parts to loosening. But the main thing is to simply focus on moving the hips. It's simple, yet we have a hard time doing it. By "it" I mean focusing.

Many of us just don't concentrate at the depth needed to move the hips in ways other than we're accustomed to. I don't blame them. I had a lot of trouble myself focusing my attention, narrowing it down to inside the hips. However, I think my tips for training the attention to do that are paying off for learners in our group who practice outside of class, as well as in class.

Eight Pieces of Brocade

I often do Eight Pieces of Brocade (*Ba Duan Jin*) after loosening as a warm-up stretching exercise. These eight postures and transitions make up a very old qigong that incorporates power stretching, spiraling, open-close, up-down, front-back, left-right and energetic realignment. It may seem to be a physical exercise at first, but it is also a *qigong*, since each move adjusts and regulates an organ, such as liver, heart, lungs, stomach, kidneys, and central nervous system. Breath is incorporated, as well.

Eight Pieces of Brocade is ultimately a path of becoming aware of *qi* and learning to move it, and directing it at will. The healing aspect of this *qigong* is its true power.

It is an energy *qigong*, in effect, because as you learn to do the postures you relax the muscles and allow energy to travel in previously unused channels. It is also a martial *qigong* because it incorporates many, if not most, of the essential configurations of tai chi internal movements (see six directions previously discussed).

There are several versions of Eight Pieces of Brocade and many barely resemble each other. I have been using Lam, Kam-Chuen's version for its simplicity when teaching beginners.

Single Basics

Single basics are rhythmic repetitions of a single pattern of movement. They are part of the repertory of techniques for training in fighting arts. What is significant about them is not so much that they are martial in nature, or originated in the process of inventing martial applications. They are actual points of entry into the framework, the edifice of learning that is *taijiquan*. They are points of practice for discovering the concepts and principles of tai chi.

By rhythmic repetition of a single pattern of movement, we create a space for our attention to notice new things about how we move and how we see movement. Through repetition of the single basics you construct a space for widening your awareness. Science knows that the human mind can concentrate on at least two things at the same time (more in reality, but we don't normally). We're born with the ability, like one of our five senses. If we were to cultivate it, it could be a basis for achieving many things that we set our intention to do.

Sooner or later, in the process of doing single basics, you become more cognizant of the muscles tensing, holding back free, fluid movement. With enough practice, meaning repetitions, you become more familiar with the difficulty of doing this, since the muscles don't automatically release. Then with more practice, you realize that it's your thinking, or your mindset, that's influencing the ability of the muscles to be in full harmony with the rest of the body in each motion.

> *Tai chi basics, such as "single-basic moves" are employed to train for specific objectives, such as loosening, relaxing and strengthening joints, ligaments and tendons, all of which are exclusive offerings of the tai chi exercise system.*

It's like learning a different language all together, a language of the body. It's a language of the whole being, in which its parts communicate with each other by virtue of an innate ability that we lose touch with as we age. A language based in feeling, observation, awareness, using all of our available senses.

What I mean is our command of language, as well as our understanding and knowledge, can limit how we describe what tai chi is. The teacher says "shoulders sit on the dantian like a boat floats on the water," but beginners don't get it automatically after hearing that instruction. We struggle to transfer the metaphor to actual practice in the moment. By doing single-basic movements, we can ultimately get the essential meaning, as well as the most practical grasp and application of "shoulder on dantian."

What I like about single basic moves is they give you something to do on your own. Good solo practice. I write before about two kinds of memory: learning a sequence of moves and remembering a deeper feeling of the movement. The latter is the "how" part of the moves.

As such, single basics are more productive ways to develop the internal.

By doing a single move at a time you give yourself a break from the process of remembering sequences. You can narrow your focus on the internal which entails deepening the attention. Not that it needs that much, just that we don't typically focus on that. We're out of touch and out of practice.

Repeating a single move simplifies the process of moving. You have less to remember. You can relax and pay more attention to the feeling of the movement and not worry so much about what comes next.

Single basics facilitate relaxation, giving you a chance someday to remain relaxed when doing more complex moves at greater speeds.

Single basic moves can help become aware of something that you were not aware of before, or haven't been for a long time. New feeling appears even when you're not actually practicing anything at all—just going through daily life.

Although single basics are "repetitive," they are not "repetitious," so to speak. You repeat a pattern intent on refining, not on repeating it exactly the same way as before. Change is the key. "Changeability" as Master Xu puts it.

How do you refine? Pick out a particular locus and focus your attention on how you move there. Focus on the move itself and how you might alter it—make it smoother, rounder, less hesitant.

You can focus also on moving along a line—from feet to head and head to feet, for example. It's like traveling along a conduit of energy. This is a more intricate view of the "flow" you hear people talk about to describe the feeling of energy moving.

For many the movement is rather broad—still more *wai dan* (external field), then *nei dan* (internal field). Both views are accurate but they have different outcomes, and different motivations.

Wai dan describes a less-informed and less-formed view, which happens to be broad in perspective. Most people begin with this mindset. *Nei dan* is deeper, revealing much more of the total scope of practice that is possible. It is deeper, less superficial.

Wherever you are in your learning process, progress happens by keeping it simple and seeking deeper awareness of what constitutes any move. Single basics is a great way to immerse yourself into this area of learning. You should be able to take greater advantage of the overall benefits of tai chi by doing single basics.

Qi and Letting Go

One of the things you notice in tai chi practice is how a particular move that you're trying to get seems harder at first, then gets easier as you practice. You wonder how it could have been so difficult. The answer is simpler than we think. "Just let go" may sound like an over simplification, but it's as easy as that.

Life force, intrinsic energy, vital energy, subtle energy. *Qi* is all of these. In more-advanced degrees of practice, *qi*, directed by mind intention moves to a point in the body and fills where you are directing your focus, such as the hamstrings or sacrum, or anywhere.

Qi flows linearly, as well as fills in all directions. Linearly, you can direct it as it sequences through the body like a string of pearls, as the old analogy goes. Practicing the microcosmic circulation *qigong* is a good way to see this and intend it in movement practice. Performing the *large* circuit, you can see it rising from the bubbling spring, up through the muscle and fascia of the legs into the hip assembly, then up to the top of the head. This tends to straighten the posture.

Microcosmic Circulation Meditation

> *"The 'Microcosmic Orbit (小周天), also known as the 'Self Winding Wheel of the Law' and the circulation of light is a Taoist Qigong or Taoist yoga Qi energy cultivation technique. It involves deep breathing exercises in conjunction with meditation and concentration techniques which develop the flow of qi along certain pathways of energy in the human body which may be familiar to those who are studying Traditional Chinese Medicine, Qigong, T'ai chi ch'uan, Neidan and Taoist alchemy."* Learn more: **https://en.wikipedia.org/wiki/Microcosmic_orbit**

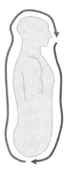

Microcosmic circulation

To briefly describe the small circuit exercise, you guide the breath to eight vessels in the body, fill them, then guide attention to the next one and fill it: *dantian*, perineum, sacrum, between shoulder blades, back of neck, crown of head, between brows, solar plexus.

If you fight against the rising—you'll crumple, collapse, or bind up. The *qi* won't flow. This points to resistance within yourself as a reluctance to let go. The *qi* makes you aware that you're holding on or closing too much.

We have to come to some clarity about this—that we hold on. Not that we're afraid to let go. Fear of *Qi* is not the problem, but we're holding and clenching out of unexamined habit. *Qi* is a healing force and when allowed to flow can reconnect the body.

Resistance, or fighting against one's own self, is very tiring physically and mentally. Wouldn't it be nice to let it all go and trust that you are made of whatever it takes to move through life without falling down, or apart?

> *Leave (some)* Qi *in the reservoir.*
> *Let breath travel.*
> *Breathing is a cooperation between qi, blood, and breath,*
> *body and mind, change and intent.*
> *Breath travels long and short*—zhong ding.
> Qi *shrinks and expands*—dantian.

Major sticking points to *qi* flowing are the hips, waist and neck. If you could move *qi* all the way from the earth through the *bai hui* (crown of head), something in these places would have to open up and let it pass. If you learn to adjust their positions (*zhong ding* or postural alignment), *qi* could suddenly flow through, and probably would.

Qi doesn't flow just linearly. When the *qi* enters the thighs, for example, it fills the thigh, causing it to expand energetically, similarly to how the lungs expand when they fill with air. You feel energy through the smallest confines of the membrane, as well as the larger areas. It's as if it even expands out of the flesh into the space beyond the body.

It wants to flow, so you change your shape to allow it to go up and it enters and fills the hips which further changes your position, maybe tilting the pelvis down and forward and up a little, then rising up the spine readjusting the vertebrae.

You either let this happen or you don't. I prefer to let it happen, but for a long time I fought against it, unaware I was holding back. This tendency reminds me of absentmindedly thinking about something or someone while I'm performing some mundane task, such as pulling weeds, taking a walk, reading or talking to another person. Then, like waking from a dream, I suddenly realize I had been in absentminded reverie while my physical body was involved in some activity I barely noticed I was doing. I don't seem to realize I'm doing it and yet there I am doing it.

Sometimes you lose the continuity in the flow. It breaks, like cutting a taut string. This is not resistance to the self, rather a sort of losing yourself and not knowing how to reconnect to the activity. This is associated with skipping the attention from one place to another. It's breaking mental concentration and deflecting your attention away from deeper levels of body awareness. This relates to being connected and whole body moves as single unit.

Another place of holding *qi* is the diaphragm. This holding is subtler than the other parts. It stems from how we breathe. The diaphragm can harden from breathing abdominally, blocking air/*qi* passing into the lower lung, then on into the upper chest. If you breathe more relaxed and less forcefully, the diaphragm can soften and become more pliable and changeable. It will function more efficiently and its range of motion will expand to its real capabilities.

As you practice you may, probably will, become cognizant of tightness in the lower back and/or the psoas muscle, as well as other places. The rope-like muscles along the lower spine may also feel quite hard to the touch. The combination of movement and breathing can soften these places and incorporate them in the overall movement with all the beneficial results that come from letting go.

Single basic moves help you to let go of tight spots, get them moving and allowing *qi* to flow. Then you can feel the *qi*, the energy of it, which feeds further practice and growth. Part of the trick of releasing is to move somewhere other than the stuck part. Single-basic moves can help accomplish this—help to recognize stuck areas where they are clenching, and having little or no *qi* flow.

Often the act of letting go takes a direction, and letting go is simply letting the muscle or ligament, tendon, bone, joint go its natural way.

Part of the release and the relief of letting go of things that are not essential to our well-being is distinguishing between what is necessary to be concerned about and what is not necessary. So the act—as simple as it may be—of letting something go, anything at all, is emancipating. Our bodies respond accordingly and become satisfied, contented, rested.

In *zhong ding* practice the idea is to let go all around and allow the *zhong ding* to provide your balance. Just sustain your focus on the *zhong ding*. *Shen* is key to doing this. With mind intention, you can evolve a more palpable sense of *zhong ding*. It becomes more real. You feel it and it begins to have an effect.

In this case we are letting go of fixations we have on the sequence of movement. Instead of moving because we want to do something, like grab a sandwich and run, we are visualizing the actual act of doing that.

Counterweight

In counterweight, you use the bones of the buttocks, legs and feet to compress and expand simultaneously, and leverage your body to move your opponent. It takes considerable amount of energy to do at first, especially when applying it in two-person practice. But it gets easier and feels good, too.

I suppose reading about this technique won't be enough to be able to actually do it in practice, but it's a beginning. Few people seem to grasp the meaning, much less know how to do it deliberately. But it's achievable when you get some hands-on exposure.

I find myself letting go of tension in the lower back in order to focus on the hip-leg-foot connectivity. An opposing power, or dynamic tension, remains throughout the move. For best effect, you must maintain connection during the switch from one direction to the other. In counterweight, you don't *float* in the transition.

With counterweight correctly implemented, it's easier to be *peng* (full, expansive) and advance the *yi* (mind), thus *qi* (energy). Also, you're outside of yourself focused on space, or imagining an opponent.

You can look at doing counterweight as drawing energy inward like a suction cup action through the feet, calves, thighs, and buttocks. Drawing up energy is similar to what Master Xu refers to as "four-become-one" posture. Suck through legs and arms into the center. Then you expand out and up until the body is the shape of an X. You are shrinking and expanding at the same time, quiet deep within, full and powerful, yet relaxed.

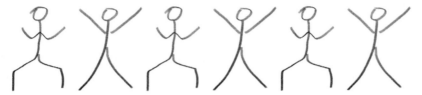

Four become one open/close exercise

It's not impossible to grasp and do, just not easy to break fixations that hinder efforts to see how to. You *can* know in an instant without trying to understand and do without hesitation or doubt, with a sense of confidence. Abandonment is a word that comes to mind in this case.

I mention counterweight here as a point of reference for your future practice. While it's difficult to transmit written instruction clearly, to be aware of its existence is essential in order to learn its significance if not an ability to actually do it. So much I discuss in *Practicing Tai Chi* is elusive in practice, but only by gaining exposure to the concepts and language can you begin to "get" it.

Stretching

I show learners a simple stretch that can do wonders to open the body and give insights into maintaining a "ready" position during movements. Using a chair, place one foot flat on the seat and stretch up straight with the leg on the ground.

Foot should be in straight line with chair. Psoas must be open, trunk straight. No leaning to the side or jutting the hip out to the side as a result of sinking into it. The ground leg must be straight, like a pole balancing on its end. It's a good idea to use another chair to steady yourself. I often touch people lightly with one finger and they are knocked off balance. That's how unbalanced they are to begin with!

Once the posture is established you can spiral left and right to feel stretching in different sections of the leg and torso.

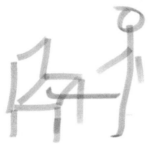

Stretch exercise

Power Stretching

Power stretching is an overlooked aspect of martial arts training, I think. Many practitioners understand tai chi as a tendon-stretching exercise, but they might not think of it as power stretching. Tai chi is much more, of course. Energetic movement is a huge part of tai chi that has informed my practice for a long time. It takes time to develop understanding of the many streams of this multi-layered practice. So getting to power stretching often is not at the top of the list for many practitioners.

When power stretching was introduced to me, I was training in *Lan Shou Men* (Blocking Hand System). My body responded well to the sets that my teachers shared. Power stretching opens up channels and lets the body breathe in fresh energy. Like opening a window on a beautiful spring day and letting fresh breezes in to replace stagnant air, power stretching moves stale *qi* out from the body's nooks and crannies.

It also strengthens the body. Combine spiraling with it for even more effective results.

Master George Xu exposed me and other students to a power stretching back in 2002 through a simple set that was qigong-like in its execution. In teaching, he still combines stretching with spiraling and internal *qigong* movement (he focuses on it in his *Complete Practice* video), but he rarely power stretches himself anymore, especially physically, because he believes that doing too much has negative effects. I agree, but I also think that some stretching is needed for many practitioners, because they simple have done so little of it in their lives. Incorporating it to some degree helps to develop a more well-rounded practice.

I first started really power stretching at Master George's China Camp in 2007 with Master Wu Ji, who gave us a set of stretches from the *Lan Shou Quan* system. And in 2009, Master Shou Guan Shun gave a group of foreign students, myself among them, his *Shin Jin Ba Gu* set from the *Lan Shou* System that we practiced several times a day for several days. I still lead this one with leaners in my classes.

You can perform the postures as gently or energetically as you want, although Master Shou makes you really put yourself into it. I videotaped that set as well in different locales in Shanghai (Richard, Shin Jin Ba Gu, 2009).

These sets, or sections of them, are very good to know and practice when you have been sitting for long periods, or have done strenuous activity for a long time. They help open your body up and clean out the stagnant energy and replace it with fresh. You can do as little as three minutes or as much as 10 minutes. You can do one set three times in a row at a time. There really is no limit to what you can benefit from adding power stretching to your daily practice.

Susan A. Matthews has posted a lot of power stretching info and learning resources on her webpages at www.taichi-secrets.com or www.susanamatthews.com. There, you can learn more about the teachers I learned from, as well. Her power stretching page contains educational content. Look for the *Lan Shou* page on her video store and scroll down to the bottom of the page and read her text about power stretching.

Spiral Training (*Chan Si Jing*)

Also known as "silk reeling," these exercises of circling and spiraling movements engage the whole body. You can loosen the joints, foster relaxation, increase efficiency, and generate whole body power. They are physical in practice as opposed to *qigong* energy movement.

I started my tai chi practice doing silk reeling exercises from the Chen Style *Taijiquan* system with Master Xu. You can get a fairly comprehensive exposure to silk reeling exercises on video with Master Xu (Richard, 2017). Zhu Tian Cai, one of the four tigers of Chen Village, is known for his teaching of *Chan Se Jing*.

Two Bodies

Another "secret" is the concept of "two bodies"; one energy and the other physical. Master Xu is my main source for knowledge about two bodies, but I think this is a universal concept. I see it as a major departure from what is conventionally referred to as "mind-body connection" that is so common in alternative modality fields.

In the two bodies concept, the mind and body really are one, and your tai chi gong is really a practice bridging and connecting the energy body and the physical body. This is a *Yin-Yang* relationship between them to say the least. Separate them as *Yin* and *Yang* separate, but still remain as one. The internal and the external refer to the energy and physical bodies.

Practice involves becoming aware of this concept, eventually distinguishing them as separate, then moving them separately at will. Cultivating greater awareness of this relationship is part of a deep learning practice of tai chi, as well as *qigong*. (See section on "internal" for more.)

CHAPTER FIVE

Thoughts on Teaching Tai Chi

To be able to share knowledge is a gift. My teacher, Master Xu, told me once to "just teach the basics." I found that teaching the basics entails amassing and organizing a vast amount of information and presenting some of it in useful and engaging ways that, hopefully, satisfies learners' needs.

A considerable amount of "thinking" goes into organizing a teaching strategy and pedagogy. It has been a continual process, a years-long progression of testing hypotheses, revising, and testing again. Fortunately, I'm enjoying myself.

However, every teacher probably encounters a moment in his journey when he feels he doesn't know how to teach. He knows he doesn't, actually, and perhaps never did. This is not surprising. It may last only an hour or two, or maybe much longer, but a time comes when what you thought you knew you were doing fizzles away under the glare of a new understanding .... that other moment that comes along in the journey of every teacher.

For me, calling people "students" or "my students" can connote a relationship of authority or superiority. It suggests that I'm better than you because I know more. It presumes a predetermined ideal or expectation that must be attained and if it isn't, you fail. This hinders us and prevents us from perceiving greater potential in our abilities.

Part of the value of tai chi for me is the ability it affords human beings to evolve more consciously, more liberated from authoritative-style teacher-student relations. Given this notion then, a simple change in terminology can serve a great purpose as it redefines our interactions. So I call you practitioners or learners.

A teacher is sensitive to subtle effects of teaching methods. If I am open to new paths of learning for myself, I am able to show new paths to others.

In teaching tai chi, the teacher should let the learner find his or her own path. They do so by striking out upon it. If you ask them to do circles, show them how you do it, but let them figure out their way to do it. They may look awkward and like they're straining, but they are trying. The only thing that matters is that they try.

Each of us passes, at some point, through stages of change—incrementally moving ever-onward through unstoppable time in a personal journey. One key to learning and "teaching" is to be humble and take the view of a beginner who knows little or nothing—only, perhaps, where to begin with your practice. One place to begin is to suspend judgment. This is a humble way.

How we come to tai chi can shape our learning. It certainly has shaped my "teaching" and what I emphasize while giving lessons. I see myself as a learner even when I am teaching. Sometimes the student is the teacher in unexpected ways and the teacher is challenged to step onto new ground and shift his idea of himself and the world around. The lines between teacher and student are blurred at these times. When this happens, student and teacher alike realize that no one ever stops being the learner.

Learning

How we take up our roles as learners influences how and what we learn, or whether we learn at all. There's always a risk of not learning. We should learn with sincerity, which comes as a measure of courage.

Are we afraid to act on "heart awareness"—accept it as a guide in our dealings with each other and our environment?

During taiji practice we critique, not criticize; not to find fault with others, but to listen to what they say and do, then feedback the meanings through our own experience.

I don't need to be better than those learning from and with me. I want them to be as good as me. If they go beyond me, then I will learn from them.

What is a positive approach to recognizing the value of the information and whether or not it works for you? It is still information and all information is good to some degree. All we can do is keep practicing. Like a Buddhist keeps sitting in meditation, a "Taijist" keeps practicing moves.

Understanding comes incrementally according to what you are prepared to take in. Every new ability is accompanied inevitably by a change in self-perception; who we think we are and what we are trying to achieve in martial art practice and in life.

Sometimes clumps of insights can strike sensitive areas of the subconscious, dragging up the detritus of a life like an anchor heaves up mud from the ocean's depths. We often react by defending the one thing we had set out to overcome when we took up learning. We indulge in the very things that we don't like about ourselves.

The teacher's job is to bring the student to a point of being able to cultivate one's own unique potential. How he or she shows us this core aspect of martial arts might not be as graceful as we would like; yet, they *have* reached a level of understanding that only self-discipline and in-depth training can give. It takes a certain quality of effort to get there. It is not just sweat or time put in, because years can pass and you still might not have cultivated authentic energy and power. It's something more. It's a listening to one's self with sincere effort and a willingness to change in the midst of the human tendency to resist change and hold on to stagnant views.

Summary

Everything I write in *Practicing Tai Chi* can be elaborated upon, but I believe the contents add useful information to a practice. It may raise questions for some, but the idea really is to stimulate questions. I think I've made it rather easy to do so. I'm not pretending to have all the answers, or even a few, but I have read little in other books about topics that I cover. I hope that this book contributes a worthy amount of information to the field of knowledge to which I have dedicated so much living.

I think *Practicing Tai Chi* offers a few key themes for practice that I haven't heard elsewhere, especially in how I express it. One is, to keep in mind that whatever or however you practice, first is to focus your attention on a locus and an activity, then sustain concentration on that. This is the core practice in my approach to learning and teaching.

Technique-wise, the process goes like this: Visualize a move before actually moving; focus attention on the point from where you want to initiate movement; the *qi* will go there in a natural response to the intention being set; the body follows, completing the three-phase progression of *see, feel, do.*

Second is that you continually try despite resistance that you may encounter. Tai chi is learning about learning. I often suggest to listen to yourself for the moves that resonate with you, remember them and do them not as hard work, but for the pleasure they bring. Nourish yourself with your practice for the sake of just doing that.

Third is focus on remembering something that resonates with you. Something simple will do if you are a beginner. Some things are easier to remember when they're simple to do, but you need to challenge yourself as well. Go beyond.

Inventories and hierarchies of knowledge that you memorize are useful to a point, but then a practitioner reaches a certain threshold where such things hold little sway over the path you travel through the as-yet discovered realms of learning. Names, directories and charts are human-made and thus can be confining. They can hinder creativity and discovery.

Dantian, for example, is significant. It is a place to begin and to return to. If it had no name, it would still have substance. You could still do something with it. Perhaps the name is good only for referencing between people who are talking about it.

Learning is a discovery of unknown things, not just what someone else already appears to know and you ascribe to. A thing is not a thing just because someone tells you it is. It becomes what it is when you discover its essence on your own through your own effort. Each of us creates new experiences as we learn and practice. We are like nodules on a tree where a new branch sprouts from the trunk. Totally unique.

It might sound funny, but for me each of us who practices tai chi with some conviction towards learning new things is a pioneer, a hunter, a frontiersman or frontierswoman, a wanderer in a new land—an unknown land—of which we can know only by entering and journeying through it. Tales told by those who have been that way before are not enough. We have to go see for ourselves.

Inspired and motivated practitioners worldwide are blazing new trails and unveiling new discoveries through their individual and shared experiences. Each new explorer on the learning path is helping to keep tai chi—this *art of internal movement*—alive, and transporting it toward new possibilities.

Resources for Practice

There is so much to say about tai chi and what it is, and why it is, or is not, for you and anyone else. I could write a blog just on this subject for a long time to come. If fact, I do! Two of them! Find them at durangotaichi.wordpress.com and at durangotaichi.com.

Check out videos at www.susanamatthews.com for follow-along practice footage. "Eight Pieces of Brocade with Susan A. Matthews" is a good start for an absolute beginner with no previous practice. The idea is to have something to practice with at home.

Websites

Chinese dictionary and translation at https://www.mdbg.net/chinese/dictionary

Durangotaichi.com

Durangotaichi.wordpress.com (Dragon Journal)

Eight Pieces of Brocade. From: http://en.wikipedia.org/wiki/Baduanjin_qigong

www.GeorgeXu.com

www.SusanAMatthews.com

Hun Yuan Qigong. http://www.hunyuantaiji.co.uk and many others. View youtube.com videos of Feng Zhi Qiang.

Videos

Richard, Paul T. Editor. "Grandmaster Wang Hao Da Neijing Training." *Masters from China Video Series*, 2011, mastersfromchina.com

Richard, Paul T. Producer. "Complete Practice with Master George Xu," *Masters from China Video Series*, 2011, mastersfromchina.com.

Garrigus, D. and Matthews, S. Producers. "Eight Pieces of Brocade with Susan A. Matthews." *Masters from China Video Series*, 2003, mastersfromchina.com.

Richard, Paul T. Producer. "Shou, Guan-Shun, Master: Shin Jin Ba Gu & Push Hands Basics." *Masters from China Video Series*, 2010, , mastersfromchina.com.

Richard, Paul T. "Tai Chi Silk Reeling and Martial Applications with George Xu." *Masters from China Video Series*, 2017, mastersfromchina.com.

Richard, Paul T. Producer. "18 Circles for Power, Mass, Speed & Freedom: Advanced Training Exercises for Martial Power with Master George Xu." *Masters from China Video Series*, 2009, mastersfromchina.com.

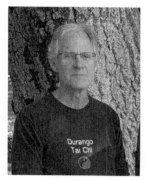

About the Author

Paul Tim Richard, MA, studies and teaches taijiquan and qigong fundamental principles. He blogs about Chinese internal martial arts and has produced instructional videos of master internal martial arts practitioners. He founded Durango Tai Chi Instruction to help others learn these arts.

Overcoming the Monster

For a long time, I was falling short of my goals and dreams, my health was compromised, I suffered from debilitating injuries that deprived me of the adventure that I expected life would be when I set out on my own. Then, luckily, I discovered a path of learning that helped to overcome those health obstacles lurking along my path. And I now have something to offer others in their search.

My quest to learn tai chi initially was in response to health challenges and as such has become a lifelong effort. Chance opportunity brought me to tai chi in 1999 after I had been learning Shotokan Karate for two years. By then, I was willing to try anything. I had been ill for a long time with back and neck injuries, as well as suffering from symptoms associated with Meniere's Disease. I was rather desperate and I didn't know what to do about it.

Physical therapists helped a little with acute conditions, but the long-term management was up to me. For the Meniere's, doctors were not helping. I got worse if anything. I eventually determined on my own that my suffering originated from deep-rooted allergies.

I'm sure I was on track to discover some sort of practice for treating these injuries and illness. But until the chance came along, I had not actually thought of tai chi as a method for healing. I probably would not have gone out of my way to find a teacher at the time.

As it happened, a work colleague who was studying with Susan Matthews leading classes in my community invited me to try it out. So I did, and that was the beginning of my journey into discovering what tai chi is and what it would mean to me.

Learning was a struggle for a few months, but I persevered long enough to be won over. I began feeling lasting results. At some point, I realized that I was overcoming my illness. Then later, I knew I would have enough control to prevent it from relapsing—just by practicing regularly and desiring to learn more. Consequently, during the following years, several teachers in China and the United States from various "internal" martial art disciplines helped me to learn by sharing some of their practices and techniques.

I learned that tai chi changes you. The study of martial arts has that effect. You set out to change a condition and in the process your practice changes you, your perspectives, your understanding, and your outlook about the meaning of health and even life itself. I'm different from the person I was when I began studying taijiquan and qigong, and other martial arts, such as xing-yi quan, lanshou quan, and bagua zhang.

Of course, some things don't change, but your self-image becomes clearer through life-long practice and study. You find yourself letting go of nonessential assumptions. Energy is freed up for more life-generating purposes.

References

This list is not nearly comprehensive, but offered merely as a place to begin.

Cohen, Kenneth S. *The Way of Qigong: The Art & Science of Chinese Energy Healing*. New York: Ballantine Books, 1997.

Davis, Barbara. *The Taijiquan Classics: An annotated translation, including a commentary by Chen Weiming*. Berkeley, CA: North Atlantic Books, 2004. Jou, Tsung Hwa. The Dao of Taijiquan: Way to Rejuvenation, 3rd Ed, Tai Chi Foundation;1989

Lam, Kam-Chuen. *The Way of Energy: Mastering the Chinese Art of Internal Strength with Chi Kung Exercise*. New York: Fireside, 1991.

Lao Tzu. *Tao Te Ching*, translated by Gia-Fu Feng and Jane English, Vintage Books, 1989, p85. There are at least 40 English translations. I suggest exploring.

Microcosmic Circuit. https://en.wikipedia.org/wiki/Microcosmic_orbit

Moyers, Bill. "The Mystery of Chi." *Healing and the Mind*, Volume 1. 1993, billmoyers.com.

Wile, Douglas, *Lost T'ai-Chi Classics from the Late Ch'ing Dynasty*, Albany, NY: State University of New York, 1996.

Yang, Jwing-Ming. *The Root of Chinese Qigong: Secrets for Health, Longevity & Enlightenment*. Wolfeboro, NH: YMAA Publications, 1997.

Zull, James E. *The Art of Changing the Brain: Enriching Teaching by Exploring the Biology of Learning*. Sterling, Virginia: Stylus Publ., 2002.

Printed in Great Britain
by Amazon